PRACTICAL GUIDE TO HEALTH ASSESSMENT

THROUGH THE LIFE SPAN

PRACTICAL GUIDE TO HEALTH ASSESSMENT

THROUGH THE LIFE SPAN

Third Edition

Mildred O. Hogstel, PhD, RN, C
Professor Emeritus
Harris School of Nursing
Texas Christian University
Fort Worth, Texas

Linda Cox Curry, PhD, RN
Professor
Harris School of Nursing
Texas Christian University
Fort Worth, Texas

F. A. Davis Company • Philadelphia

F. A. Davis Company
1915 Arch Street
Philadelphia, PA 19103
www.fadavis.com

Printed in Canada

Last digit indicates print number: 10 9 8 7 6 5 4 3 2 1

Acquisitions Editor: Lisa A. Biello
Developmental Editor: Diane Blodgett
Production Editor: Jessica Howie Martin
Cover Designer: Louis J. Forgione

As new scientific information becomes available through basic and clinical
research, recommended treatments and drug therapies undergo changes.
The authors and publisher have done everything possible to make this
book accurate, up to date, and in accord with accepted standards at the
time of publication. The authors, editors, and publisher are not responsible for errors or omissions or for consequences from application of the
book, and make no warranty, expressed or implied, in regard to the contents of the book. Any practice described in this book should be applied
by the reader in accordance with professional standards of care used in regard to the unique circumstances that may apply in each situation. The
reader is advised always to check product information (package inserts)
for changes and new information regarding dose and contraindications
before administering any drug. Caution is especially urged when using
new or infrequently ordered drugs.

Library of Congress Cataloging-in-Publication Data

Hogstel, Mildred O.
    Practical guide to health assessment through the life span /
Mildred O. Hogstel, Linda Cox Curry.—3rd ed.
        p. cm.
    Includes bibliographical references and index.
    ISBN 0-8036-0803-9 (pbk.)
    1. Nursing assessment—Handbooks, manuals, etc. I. Curry, Linda
Cox. II. Title.

RT48.H643 2001
616.07′5—dc21

                                                    2001017246

To Our Families
and Students

Preface

Health assessment is an essential component of the nursing process and includes the health history; psychosocial history; physical, functional, and mental status examinations; and cultural, ethnic, family, and environmental assessments. The essential components of the assessment process may be completed in a few minutes in an emergency; at the other extreme, assessment may take place over several weeks in the client's home. The nurse has to use judgment in deciding which parts of the assessment are needed for a specific client in a certain setting depending on priorities.

The purpose of this book is to provide nursing students and practicing nurses in all areas including community settings with a practical and easy-to-use reference to the major components, sequence, and methodology of health assessment. It is assumed that the user of this book will have completed courses in anatomy and physiology and will have completed or currently be enrolled in a course in health assessment.

This book can easily be kept in a pocket until needed. When the nurse is ready to perform any part of the assessment, the book may be placed on a table near the client's bed or chair. The book has been designed for easy reference. The third edition has been expanded to include more content that will be helpful in better understanding the assessment process. New areas include assessment of the use of alternative and complementary therapies; antepartum and intrapartum assessment; expanded coverage of communication skills, especially when communicating with clients of different ages, with different needs, and from different cultural and ethnic backgrounds; family communication and assessment; variations in physical assessment based on various racial and ethnic differences; and a basic orientation to and expansion of physical assessment techniques. The equipment needed, sequence, and techniques for each system have also been expanded. The steps of what to assess in carrying out a physical examination of each body system are listed. It should be noted that some of the assessment techniques (for example, an internal gynecologic examination and a prostate examination) are included as essential components of a total assessment, but they will not be performed by the novice practitioner.

Normal and/or common findings and *significant deviations* from normal are included for each system. *Common* findings are those that are not considered *normal* because they do not occur in everyone but that rarely need referral (e.g., lentigo senilis in older adults or cradle cap in infants). *Common* and *significant* findings that should be referred for follow-up are shown in color. A special section, clinical alert, is also in color. This section notes special instructions the nurse needs to be aware of during the assessment and/or concerns related to the findings such as immediate referral.

A few sample diagnostic tests are listed for each system. The nurse will refer the client to a physician, advance practice nurse (where appropriate), or other healthcare provider who may order and evaluate the diagnostic tests. Sample North American Nursing Diagnosis Association (NANDA) nursing diagnoses are also included for each system. These are not meant to be inclusive because nursing diagnoses are very individualized. However, the samples should guide the reader toward other possible diagnoses. These diagnoses should be helpful in preparing individual care plans after the assessment phase. Essential client and family education, home health notes, and a list of associated community agencies for each system also have been expanded or added.

Perinatal, pediatric, and geriatric adaptations have been revised for each section of the health history, physical examination, and client-family education. Racial and ethnic adaptations and additions have been made where appropriate. For each body system, a brief sample of how to document the physical findings is presented. Samples of primarily *normal* and some *common abnormal* findings are documented. *Significant deviations* from normal will need more detailed documentation. These samples are only a general guide because methods of documentation vary with the institution or agency format, the setting, and the client's needs or status.

The appendices contain selected sample history, mental status, functional assessment, and physical assessment forms as well as other reference material that will be helpful in performing and documenting a complete health assessment. A glossary of the most commonly used abbreviations and terms in health assessment appears at the back of the book so that other references will not be needed for this information. Following this is a list of specific references used in each of the three sections of the book and other health assessment resources that may be consulted for further reading.

The authors believe that nurses will find this assessment book a helpful, time-saving clinical guide while they are learning or becoming more skilled in health assessment techniques in the classroom or any clinical setting in which they assess clients.

Mildred O. Hogstel
Linda Cox Curry

Acknowledgements

The authors express their appreciation to the contributors for their helpful additions, and to Susan Moore, Executive Assistant, for typing the manuscript.

Contributors

Pediatric Adaptations by

Marinda Allender, RN, MSN
Instructor
Harris School of Nursing
Texas Christian University
Fort Worth, Texas

Geriatric Adaptations by

Katy Scherger, RN, MSN, CS
Gerontological Nurse Practitioner
Evercare
Tucson, Arizona

Communication Additions Including Cultural/Ethnic Adaptations and Home Care, Teaching, Documentation, and Community Resources by

Danna Strength, DNSc, RN
Associate Professor
Harris School of Nursing
Texas Christian University
Fort Worth, Texas

General and Intrapartum Physical Assessment by

Mary Beth Walker, RN, MS
Instructor
Harris School of Nursing
Texas Christian University
Fort Worth, Texas

Contents

PART 1

1 The Client Interview and Health History

Contents
continued

List of Figures

List of Tables

The Client Interview and Health History

CHAPTER 1
OVERVIEW OF THE NURSING PROCESS

The profession of nursing is made up of many roles and activities. Several scholars and theorists have defined the profession of nursing, but the most commonly accepted definition is the one offered in 1980 by the American Nurses' Association (ANA): "the diagnosis and treatment of human responses to actual or potential health problems." This means that nurses care for people, as individuals or groups, who are reacting to actual health problems. Additionally, nurses attempt to prevent problems and promote maintenance in people who are healthy.

The framework for nursing practice is the *nursing process,* which is an organized problem-solving method. The nursing process was defined and refined in the 1950s to 1970s. It is made up of five sequential steps: assessment, diagnosis, planning, implementation, and evaluation. Through application of the nursing process, the nurse is able to deliver nursing care, for example, to diagnose and treat human responses to health problems.

The nursing process also provides a common language for nurses to use in any geographic area or specialty practice. The ANA developed its standards of care around the nursing process, and the licensing examination is structured to test knowledge of the five steps in the process. The focus of this text is on the first step of the nursing process, assessment. The steps are briefly explained in the next section.

Assessment is focused on the collection of information about the client and the client's problem(s) in order to lay a foundation for the remainder of the process. Data may be *subjective*, that is, perceived only by the client, or it may be *objective*, that is, able to be validated by the nurse or other health-care professional. Examples of subjective data include nausea, pain, and feelings of worthlessness. Examples of objective data include vomiting, facial expressions and physical behaviors, and laboratory data. Subjective data are most often collected during the nursing history, usually an interview. Objective data may be observed at any time but are most often collected during the physical examination or review of the medical record for laboratory or other findings.

The second step is *nursing diagnosis* and consists of clustering and organizing the data gathered during assessment. The data that fit together into a diagnosis category are then labeled with a diagnosis that guides the remainder of the nursing process. The diagnosis not only organizes the data but also provides a fast and articulate description of the client's problems or needs. These nursing diagnoses are widely available and are reviewed annually by the North American Nursing Diagnosis Association (NANDA). Refer to Appendix A for the most current list of nursing diagnoses.

The third step in the nursing process is *planning*. This step has several components including (a) placing the diagnoses in priority order, (b) identifying outcome criteria to facilitate evaluation, (c) identifying the nursing interventions necessary to reach the outcomes, and (d) documenting of this step in the appropriate place and manner for the institution or agency. Planning is accomplished with the help of the client and family and is essential to the smooth delivery of care.

Implementation is the fourth step in the process. Using the plan as a guide, the nurse carries out the plan and communicates with other staff and the client. In this step, the nurse may be teaching a new parent how to bathe a baby, an older adult how to inject a medication, or a family member how to change a dressing on a surgical wound. This step also includes the documentation of care in the client record.

The fifth and final step of the nursing process is *evaluation.* In this step, the nurse assesses the client's progress toward the outcomes identified in the planning process. If revisions in the care plan are necessary, they should be instituted. If the outcome has been reached, the problem is resolved. The evaluation step generates new assessment data, and the process continues.

The nursing process can be illustrated in the care of a client on the first day after abdominal surgery and the activities involved in only one problem. The nurse collects the following data during assessment: The client is crying and asking for pain relief; there is an 8-inch surgical incision across her lower abdomen; the client is restless and guarding the incision during movement, and the client has had no pain medication for 6 hours. A diagnosis of acute pain would guide the nurse toward suggested interventions such as providing comfort measures, administering medications, and encouraging family support. The planning phase includes proposed interventions and such details as how much medication to give and how often it can be given. For example, after the client experienced relief, the nurse would plan to teach about pain management, including the timing of medications. The planning phase also includes identifying outcome criteria to guide evaluation methods such as assessing the client's ability to sleep or function, as well as asking the client to describe the level of pain relief. The implementation phase is the administration of medications, positioning the client with pillows under the abdomen, and teaching about pain. This step also includes documenting the assessment data, nursing actions, and responses of the client in the record. The last step is evaluation. In this example, the nurse would assess the client's pain relief by asking the client to rank the level of pain, as well as observing the client's behavior, as observed by the ability to sleep or a relaxed facial expression.

To be effective, the nursing process requires significant knowledge and skills. For example, the nurse must have an understanding of physiology, psychology, chemistry, and nutrition to identify obesity in an adolescent and develop a plan of care. The nurse must have adequate skills to conduct a thorough assessment, such as auscultating breath sounds or describing a skin lesion. Finally, the nurse must have psychomotor skills to carry out activities such as diapering a newborn or inserting an intravenous catheter.

The purpose of this text is to assist the nurse in developing and mastering the skills and knowledge associated with the assessment phase of the nursing process. These include communication and technical skills based on a broad background in the sciences and humanities.

CHAPTER 2
COMMUNICATION SKILLS

Effective communication is an essential component of the total nursing process. How a nurse speaks to, listens to, looks at, responds to, and touches a person often determines how that person will share information, thoughts, and feelings and cooperate with the plan of care. Most clients can tell by the nurse's first contact and approach what kind of relationship is likely to develop. Clients can usually tell if nurses are interested in them by the way they speak, stand, or sit and listen, as well as what they say.

Attentive listening is one of the most important skills a nurse can develop. And, it is not as easy as it sounds. Attentive listening—hearing what the other person is saying and understanding the meaning of words, gestures, and mannerisms—during a 1-hour session with a client can be much more tiring and difficult than speaking for an hour.

EFFECTIVE COMMUNICATION

Effective *communication* is essential for successfully *interviewing* the client to obtain his or her health history:

- Communication may be defined as one's attempt to understand another person's point of view from his or her frame of reference.
- Interviewing may be defined as conversation directed by the nurse for the explicit purpose of seeking information from the client. It includes the use of verbal and nonverbal behavior by the nurse to communicate with the client.
- Communication is used in every intervention with the client from the time of admission and the taking of a health history through discharge planning and teaching home-health-care needs.

Effective communication, although often time consuming, can enhance nursing care and possibly prevent problems later. When nurses develop trusting and open relationships with clients early in their care, the clients are usually more open, more cooperative, and less likely to complain or be upset if everything does not go as planned later.

Purposes of Therapeutic Communication

The purposes of therapeutic communication are to

- Exchange ideas, information, feelings
- Understand another person's point of view
- Understand another person's frame of reference
- Assist in establishing the nurse-client relationship
- Effect change in nurse-client situations
- Disseminate information
- Assist in clarifying problems

Aspects of Each Message

- What the sender wants to convey
- What the sender conveys
- What the receiver hears
- What the receiver thought he or she heard

5

- How the receiver interprets the message (see Fig. 2–1)

The aspects of each message are influenced by barriers or factors that can affect the communication process. These include

- Individual qualities of each participant (beliefs, needs, values, sociocultural background, age, gender, and current physical and emotional status)
- Capacity of sender and receiver to speak and hear
- Relationship between sender and receiver
- Purpose of the communication
- Content of message being sent
- Setting and/or environmental conditions and distractions (setting may be unfamiliar to client, which can cause anxiety)
- Previous experiences associated with the present situation
- Language skill of interviewer

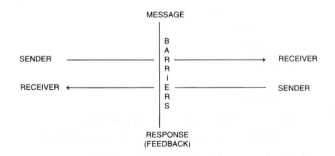

FIGURE 2–1
Components of communication.

Criteria for Effective Verbal Communication

- <u>Brevity:</u> Get to the point.
- <u>Clarity:</u> Avoid ambiguous words and generalizations.
- <u>Simplicity:</u> Use lay terms and avoid medical terminology.
- <u>Timing and relevancy:</u> Send message when it needs to be sent in relation to the client's interests and concerns.

REMEMBER

<u>It is impossible not to communicate.</u> When one is not using <u>verbal</u> communication, it must be remembered that <u>nonverbal</u> communication is occurring. Nonverbal communication is the exchange of messages without the use of words.

Nonverbal Communication

- Body language (for example, use of hands or arms)
- Facial expressions
- Eye contact (depends on culture)
- Lip movements
- Gestures
- Posture
- Physical appearance (including clothes and grooming)
- Space (distance between two people)
- Touch (differentiate for skilled care and support)
- Silence (can be therapeutic or awkward)
- Qualities of voice (intonation, rate, rhythm, pitch)
- Active listening

Guidelines for Active and Effective Listening

- Avoid interruptions.
- Concentrate on the speaker.
- Maintain eye contact if culturally appropriate to do so.
- Lean toward and face the speaker.
- Maintain open posture, not crossed arms.
- Make a conscious effort to hear and <u>understand</u> the other person; avoid premature interpretations and judgments.
- Avoid extensive note taking.

Guidelines for Use of Touch

Touch is a form of nonverbal communication that is a learned behavior filled with meaning. Touch is generally not necessary in obtaining a health history but is necessary in performing a physical assessment. This poses a difficult problem for the nurse. In general, it is best to avoid the use of touch, particularly invasive procedures, until a nurse-client relationship is well established and the nurse is knowledgeable about the beliefs related to touch in the particular culture. When touch becomes necessary, it is best used by members of the same gender and culture. If touch seems appropriate while taking a nursing history (e.g., if a client should begin crying), gentle touch of the nurse's hand on the client's upper arm or shoulder could be used. Touch will be covered under each of the cultural groups in the cultural variation section.

DEVELOPMENTAL CONSIDERATIONS IN COMMUNICATION

Age and gender are factors to consider when communicating with clients. The nurse does not communicate with a 5-year-old, a 45-year-old, or a 95-year-old in the same manner. Although the nurse should be himself or herself in each individual situation, variations in approach will be needed. For example, motherspeak (baby talk) is not appropriate past a certain age, and it should not be assumed that all 95-year-old people have a hearing deficit.

Infants

- Address the baby by given name.
- Do not address parents as "Mom" or "Dad."
- Speak to the infant before beginning assessment.

Toddlers

- Introduce yourself.
- Spend time talking to parent before approaching child.
- Allow parent to remain close to child.
- Have stuffed animal or toy for child to play with.
- Sit at eye level to child.

Preschoolers

- Introduce yourself.
- Call the child by name.
- Ask the child simple questions directly.
- Allow child to manipulate equipment before using it on child.
- Sit at eye level to child.

School-Age Children

- Address questions concerning habits and health promotion to the child.
- Encourage the child rather than the parent to answer.
- Provide explanations of assessment techniques as well as findings.
- Provide health teaching directly to the child.

Adolescents

- Obtain some preliminary history information from adolescent and parent.
- Then ask to speak to adolescent alone.
- Discuss confidential issues with adolescent.
- Use open-ended questions ("Tell me about . . . ," "Many teenagers are concerned about . . .").
- Listen and respond in a nonthreatening or non-judgmental manner.

Adults*

- Always face the person and establish eye contact.
- Speak slowly and clearly. Watch your accent.
- Always respect the rights and dignity of the person.
- Do not use complicated medical terminology.
- Use common lay terminology without being overly simplistic.
- Let the person set the pace of the conversation.
- Do not interrupt the person.
- Do not crowd the person unless you are invited or encouraged to come close.
- Avoid distracting body signals like finger tapping and seat shifting.
- Try not to appear distracted by unseemly or grotesque appearances or uncontrolled gestures.
- If you do not speak his or her language well, do not try at all, but get an interpreter or signer.
- Assume nothing.
- Sit if the person is sitting or lying down.

*Source: Adapted from material provided by the Long-term Care Ombudsman Program of the Mental Health Association of Tarrant County.

- Always regard what the person has to say as important.
- Be kind and warm, but firm.
- Make no promises you cannot keep.
- Under some circumstances, silent presence can be very comforting and reassuring and can be a strong statement of concern and care.

Older Adults* (See also App. B)
Preparation

- Always introduce yourself by your full name and explain your role unless the person knows you by name or recognition.
- Never patronize an older person. Greet the person by Mr., Mrs., Miss, Ms., or Dr. and surname unless the person asks you to use another name.
- Always respect the rights and dignity of the person.
- Do not make promises you cannot keep. Be honest and direct.
- Allow time to cultivate a trusting relationship.
- Let the person set the pace of the conversation. Fight the impulse to talk rather than listen.
- Always regard what the person has to say as important.
- Be dependable. Promise only what you can control.
- Be honest. Avoid giving false hope or stating platitudes.

---

*Source: Written by Mildred O. Hogstel, Ph.D., R.N., C. (with suggestions from Ann Reban, M.S.N., R.N., C., Anne L. Lind, M.S.N., R.N., and Monnette Graves, M.S.N.).

General

- Identify yourself by name (do not be disappointed if some forget). Repeat as needed.
- Call the person by the preferred name (use first name <u>only</u> if it is preferred).
- Avoid current slang and/or filler words (e.g., "you know; it's like, cool, man").
- Keep yourself in the person's view so that he or she can see your face. (Talking at the side or in the back may cause difficulty with communication and confusion.)
- Use direct eye contact. Sit or stand at the same level as the person.
- Use a calm, clear, slightly slower, lower-pitched voice. Do not speak loudly or shout because this can cause auditory discomfort.
- Speak louder only if you are sure the person has a hearing loss. (Check if you are uncertain.)
- Try not to sound angry if you must speak loudly.
- Repeat if necessary. Speak once the same way; if you are still not understood, rephrase.
- Eliminate background noise (e.g., television).
- Ask one question at a time and wait for a response.
- Allow time for responses. It may take a little longer than you expect.
- Do not interrupt the person because doing so discourages responses.
- <u>Listen attentively.</u>

Written

- Name tags with large type and category of personnel are helpful.

- Use written notes as reminders (e.g., names of family and friends).
- Label names of people on pictures.

Body Language

- Use an open, gentle approach and genuine smile.
- Use a gentle touch. (A gentle pat on the hand can test the person's response.)
- Evaluate acceptability of hugs. Response to touch and protection of personal space vary among individuals.
- A simple nod of the head is appropriate.

COMMUNICATING WITH PEOPLE WHO ARE PHYSICALLY CHALLENGED*

Communicating with the Hearing Impaired

- Find out if the person has a hearing aid.
- If the person wears a hearing aid and still has difficulty hearing, check to see if the hearing aid is in the person's ear, turned on, adjusted, and has a working battery.
- Wait until you are directly in front of the person, you have the person's attention, and you are close to the person before you begin speaking.
- Be sure that the person sees you as you approach her or him.
- Always face the hard-of-hearing person. Be on the same level with the person whenever possible and gain eye contact.
- Do not chew gum or smoke, and keep your hands away from your face while talking.

---

*Source: Adapted from material provided by the Long-term Care Ombudsman Program of the Mental Health Association of Tarrant County.

- Speak slowly and clearly.

- Do not let your voice trail or drop off at the end of a sentence or phrase.

- Never shout. Shouting distorts sound and turns word symbols into noise.

- Reduce background noises as much as possible when carrying on a conversation.

- Use simple, short sentences to make your conversation easier to understand.

- Do frequent checks to see if the person is understanding you.

- Write messages if necessary. Ask relatives how they communicate with the person.

- Do not be impatient. Allow ample time to converse with a hearing-impaired person. Being in a rush will compound everyone's stress and create barriers to having a meaningful conversation.

Communicating with the Deaf

Communicating with people who are deaf is similar to communicating with the hearing impaired.

- Ask relatives or friends of the deaf person how they communicate.

- Write messages if the person can read.

- Use devices with illustrations (e.g., a picture board, as shown in Fig. 2–2), to facilitate communication.

- Be concise with your statement and questions.

- Allow sufficient time to visit with the person.

- Face the person when speaking.

Communicating with the Visually Impaired

- Touch is important. You might offer your hand, or if you are walking, offer use of your arm as guidance.

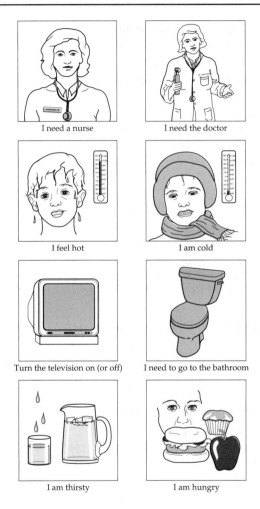

FIGURE 2–2

These drawings can be used with any client who has expressive or receptive deficits related to communications (e.g., hearing deficit, language disorder, or other barriers). Thanks to Joey Eckstein for the original sketches from which these figures were prepared.

- Call out the person's name before touching. Touching lets a person know you are listening.
- Allow the person to touch you.
- Tell the person if you are leaving. Let the person know if others will remain in the room or if she or he will be alone.
- If you are in a group, always begin your comments by saying the name of the person to whom you are addressing.
- Treat the visually impaired person as you would a fully sighted individual. This will help the person you are talking with feel at ease and confident.
- Find out from the individual the extent of her or his impairment. Legal blindness is not necessarily total blindness.
- Use the words <u>see</u> and <u>look</u> normally.
- Explain what you are doing, as you are doing it.
- Encourage familiarity and independence whenever possible.
- Do not be overprotective.
- Be careful not to move things around in the room of a visually impaired person unless the person asks you to move something.

Communicating with Aphasics

Aphasia is a total or partial loss of the power to use or understand words. It is often the result of a stroke or other brain damage.

- Get the person's attention. Try to make sure there are no other distractions in the immediate area.
- Be patient, communicate only one idea at a time, and allow plenty of time. Speak slowly.
- Use simple, concrete adult language. Use short phrases.

- Be honest with the person. Do not pretend to understand a person when you do not.
- Allow the aphasic to try to complete thoughts, to struggle with words. Avoid being too quick to guess what the person is trying to express.
- Encourage the person to write the word he or she is trying to use and read it out loud.
- Use of gestures or pointing to objects might be helpful.
- Use touch to aid in concentration, communication, reassurance, and encouragement.

COMMUNICATING WITH PEOPLE WHO ARE COGNITIVELY CHALLENGED

- Help the person to feel safe and secure.
- Ask simple yes or no questions. Speak slowly.
- Use positive statements. Help the person understand what you want him or her to do.
- Always assume that the person has the capacity to understand.
- If the person is having trouble communicating an idea, help with the word he or she is trying to find. Do not interrupt or appear impatient.
- Write down positive or reassuring information. Avoid giving information that may produce anxiety. Timing is important.
- Use short, clear, and concrete statements, one step at a time. Give step-by-step instructions.
- Do not correct mistakes made by the confused person.

COMMUNICATING WITH AGGRESSIVE PEOPLE

- Speak softly. Be calm and reassuring.
- Avoid quick, sudden, or erratic movements.
- Never argue or try to reason with the person.
- Be empathetic.
- Keep out of striking distance.
- Never threaten verbally or strike back; this is abuse.
- Avoid cornering the person. Keep a clear pathway out of the room.

CULTURAL VARIATIONS IN COMMUNICATION AND INTERVIEWING

When nurses communicate with clients from cultures different from their own, the likelihood of miscommunication increases dramatically. There are major problems in verbal communication; however, there are as many pitfalls, if not more, in nonverbal transcultural communication.

General Guidelines for Transcultural Therapeutic Communication

- Maintain an open attitude.
- Speak in a clear, slow manner.
- RRS: Restate, reflect, and summarize.
- Write important information, using drawings and pictures to increase understanding.
- Seek an interpreter when needed:
  - Identify language used at home.
  - Meet with interpreter before interview.
  - Request detailed account of the conversation.
  - Allow extra time for the interview (Jarvis, 2000).

- Avoid interpreters of a rival tribe or nation.
- The interpreter must have cultural sensitivity.
- An interpreter of the same gender is preferred.

- Recognize the influence of religion in developing beliefs, values, and healing practices.
- Develop insight into your own attitudes, beliefs, and values.
- Avoid using your own values to judge others.
- Respect the client's beliefs and values.
- Develop understanding of the role of the nuclear and extended families.
- Develop knowledge of cultural health beliefs, practices, and healers.
- Recognize that folk healing or traditional medicine may be practiced along with Western medicine.
- Avoid cultural stereotypes.

REMEMBER

Generalizations should not be applied to all members of a specific cultural or ethnic group. Communication with each client should be individualized.

Concepts that Vary by Culture and Ethnicity*
Touch

- Conveys various meanings.
- Same-gender health-care provider may be preferred.

Source: Adapted from Jarvis, C (ed): Physical Examination. Saunders, Philadelphia, 2000; and Kozier, B, Erb, G, Blais, K, Wilkinson, JM, & Van Leuven, K (eds): Fundamentals of Nursing, ed. 5. Addison-Wesley, Menlo Park, CA, 1998.

- Parental permission may be needed to touch a child.

Eye Contact

- Varies greatly among cultures (e.g., looking at the floor, downcast eyes).
- Conveys different meanings.

Space

- Value placed on space differs (e.g., territoriality).
- Size of one's intimate zone varies.
- Explain need for entry into intimate or personal space.

Time

- Values about past, present, and future vary.
- Values on promptness vary (e.g., following a time schedule).

Silence

- Uncomfortable for some.
- May convey understanding, respect, or agreement.

Formality/Informality

- Varies from expectations of an authoritarian approach of the health-care professional to a close personal relationship.

CHAPTER 3
HEALTH HISTORY GUIDELINES

See Appendix C for a sample health history form.

INTRODUCTION

Taking the client's health history serves a variety of purposes. First, the history provides the client's perspective of the database and the context of beliefs and values in which the client operates. It communicates not only the client's words but also the client's nonverbal language and inflections of voice. Second, taking the history offers an opportunity to establish rapport with the client. The interviewer can demonstrate interest in the client and the health condition and can encourage trust through both verbal and nonverbal behaviors. Third, the history provides essential direction for the remainder of the examination. For example, the client may describe a pattern of chronic alcohol abuse, which should guide the examiner in examining the liver and skin and indicate specific laboratory tests to pursue.

The client is the most important source of data for both the health history and the physical examination. Sufficient time should be allowed so that the client does not feel rushed and so that vital clues are not overlooked. Interviewing skills are improved with practice, and most nurses develop an interaction style with which they are comfortable. The nurse may occasionally need to review principles of therapeutic communication to enhance these skills.

In the case of a child or of an older client with a family member present, taking the history is an important time to include the family's data. The nurse can indicate the importance of the client as the center of the nursing process, while acknowledging the value of the family's contribution. This may also be an opportunity to observe and/or explore such family problems as caregiver stress, inadequate parenting skills, insufficient social support, or even physical or psychological abuse.

TIPS FOR INTERVIEWING

- Sit facing the client, if possible, so that the client can see your face. Sitting suggests relaxation and indicates that time will be allowed for the interview.

- Provide privacy, and attend to client comfort; for example, supply pillows for support, a footstool, or a glass of water.

- Use simple language at first; increase complexity if client is able to understand. Avoid scientific and professional jargon. Avoid condescension and patronizing tones.

- Explain the purpose of the interview, how long it will last, and how the information will be used.

- Take brief notes. Avoid emphasizing the notes but capture important statements accurately.

- Use open-ended questions such as "How do the headaches begin?" to explore feelings and perceptions and to identify areas requiring follow-up.

- Use narrow questions to help the client focus, such as "Do you have nausea with the vomiting?"

- Follow up critical areas during the initial interview. For example, a client explains that he takes digoxin and has had nausea and vomiting for 3 days. Also, record those areas that need further exploration at a later date. For example, an adolescent client reports that her grandmother has osteoporosis and uterine cancer.

- Unless contraindicated by the client's cultural background, look and listen carefully for clues, both verbal and nonverbal. Establish eye contact, avoid answering for the client, and explore clues in a nonthreatening manner.

- Avoid interruptions and the appearance of being distracted or bored, such as looking at the clock or flipping pages in the record. Wait for answers. Silence encourages thinking and often produces verbal responses.

- Avoid tiring the client. A thorough history may take from 20 minutes to 1 hour, the length varying according to the client's condition and the setting.

INTERVIEWING

Purpose of an Interview

- To establish rapport
- To establish or maintain nurse-client relationship
- To obtain information
- To identify or clarify problems
- To give information to the client or to teach him or her
- To counsel and/or assist the client in finding solutions to problems

Structure of the Interview

- <u>Directive:</u> One that is highly structured, through which specific information is sought
- <u>Nondirective:</u> One in which interviewer clarifies statements and encourages elaboration to assist client in reaching conclusions

Guidelines for an Effective Interview

- Utilize therapeutic communication.
- Identify the needed information before the interview.
- Minimize distractions in the environment.
- Use vocabulary understandable to the client.
- Be tactful about asking questions of a personal nature. Ask yourself, "Is this information really necessary?" If necessary, explain to client why the information is needed.
- Be an active listener. (See guidelines for being an active and effective listener on page 8.)

- Remain alert for answers that may be socially acceptable but not entirely accurate or for answers the client thinks the nurse wants to hear.

- Avoid rushing the client; allow time for thought. (This is especially important in cultures where periods of silence are valued.)

- Avoid letting personal beliefs, biases, or values interfere.

- Conduct interview at eye level with client.

- Look and listen for cues (e.g., changes in facial expression or posture) for follow-up questions.

- Ask nonleading, open-ended questions.

- Use an amplifying device (for example, have the client put the ear pieces of a stethoscope in his or her ears while you speak into the diaphragm, or use other assistive device) for persons with decreased hearing function.

- Avoid following a form too closely and taking extensive notes during the interview.

- Document information clearly and succinctly as soon as possible after leaving the room.

- Use direct quotes of the client when they are especially meaningful.

- Complete the interview in less than 20 minutes if you are in an acute care setting.

- At the end ask, "Is there anything else you would like to tell me?"

REMEMBER
- Summarize the interview for the client to be sure the information is correct.
- Practice interviewing to develop your skills.

INFORMATION NEEDED FOR A COMPLETE HEALTH HISTORY

The assessment begins with the complete health history. This phase helps develop rapport with the client so that he or she will feel more comfortable during the rest of the assessment. It also alerts the health-care provider about which systems and symptoms need to be assessed carefully later in the assessment process. Statements may be used such as "I am going to be asking you some questions about your past health history so we can better determine your current needs and care." All of the previously discussed content related to communication skills and interviewing techniques are especially important during this phase of the assessment. Most health-care institutions and agencies have their own history forms on which to record these data. A list of important information to obtain follows.

Date of History
Personal Data

- Name
- Gender
- Date of birth
- Place of birth
- Age
- Ethnic background
- Native language
- Marital status
- Address
- Phone number
- Name and telephone number of primary care physician (specialists if needed)
- Hospital preferred
- Social Security number
- Medicare and/or Medicaid number

- Other insurance name and number
- Religious preference, including church or synagogue membership
- Person to be contacted in an emergency (name, relationship, address, phone number)
- Education
- Occupation (presently or before retirement)

Reason for Seeking Health Care (Chief Complaint (CC))
History of Present Illness (PI)

- Onset
- Location of symptoms
- Chronology
- Setting
- Precipitating factors
- Alleviating factors
- Aggravating factors
- Associated symptoms
- Treatments
- Client's view of cause

Past Health History

- Client's perception of level of health in general
- Childhood illnesses (dates and types)
- Genogram (family history of diseases)
- Immunizations (see App. H)
- Allergies
- Serious accidents and/or injuries (dates)
- Major adult illnesses (types and dates)
- Behavioral problems
- Surgical procedures (types and dates)

- Other hospitalizations (types and dates)
- Obstetric history
- Date of menopause
- Environmental hazards:
  - Home
  - Work
  - Community
- Blood transfusions (given or received, dates)

Current Medications

- Ask client to list all prescription medications he or she is taking.
- Ask client about his or her understanding of the reasons medications were prescribed.
- Ask client to list the over-the-counter (OTC) preparations he or she is taking. The use of alternative and complimentary substances (e.g., herbs and large doses of multiple vitamins) is greatly increasing. Some interact with prescription medications and cause serious side effects. Record the names and doses of all such substances currently being taken.
- Ask client about home remedies he or she is using.
- Ask client if he or she is taking any borrowed medications.
- Ask client if he or she is experiencing any side and adverse effects from any of the medications he or she is taking. Explain the difference between side and adverse effects.
- Assess discrepancies between prescribed frequency and dose and actual pattern of intake.
- Ask to see all medications being taken. Have the client bring his or her medication to clinic, or check medications during each home visit.

- Instruct client to flush discontinued or expired medication.

- Instruct client in use of a medication organizer, which can be bought at a drugstore or made from an egg carton. For home health clients check the organizer each visit and fill prn.

- Provide a Medication Card (see App. BB) and help the client complete it so that the needed information will always be available when seeking medical care.

Personal Habits and Patterns of Living

- <u>Work:</u> Type, length of time employed, stresses
- <u>Rest and/or sleep:</u> How much, when, aids
- <u>Exercise and/or ambulation:</u> How much, when, aids
- <u>Recreation, leisure, hobbies:</u> Type, amount
- <u>Nutrition:</u> Time, foods, fluids, and amounts for all meals (24-hour recall) and snacks; recent changes in appetite; special diet
- <u>Caffeine:</u> Source, amount, problems caused by
- <u>Alcohol and/or other drugs:</u> Type, number of years used, amount, perceived problems with level of use
- <u>Tobacco:</u> Type, number of years used, amount per day
- <u>Urinary and bowel activity:</u> Frequency, amount, problems
- <u>Sexual activity:</u> Level of activity, use of contraceptives, problems, sexual orientation

Activities of Daily Living

Ask about the client's ability to perform (alone or with help) the following activities:

- Ambulating
- Dressing

- Grooming
- Bathing
- Toileting
- Eating
- Using the telephone
- Doing laundry
- Housekeeping
- Obtaining access to the community
- Driving
- Purchasing food
- Preparing food
  (See also functional assessment on page 33.)

PSYCHOSOCIAL HISTORY

The psychosocial history is important in any assessment that considers a holistic view of the client, especially in a community or long-term care setting. The psychosocial history involves the client's relationship to others such as family members, friends, neighbors, church groups, colleagues at work, and friends in social and civic organizations in the community. Assessing factual data about the client's social network and needs is essential, but determining feelings about those contacts and needs is also important. Expression of feelings is more difficult for some clients than others, but the skillful nurse who communicates well will more likely set an environment where important feelings will be expressed.

Inquire about and document the following:

- Significant others, relationship, proximity
- Support systems needed and available:
  - <u>Informal:</u> Family, friends, neighbors
  - <u>Formal:</u> Temporary Aid to Needy Families (TANF), Medicaid, Medicare, Women, Infants, Children (WIC), Food Stamps, Supplemental Security Income (SSI)

- <u>Semiformal:</u> School, church, clubs
- Satisfaction with social contacts
- Typical 24-hour weekday and weekend day:
  - Satisfaction with employment
  - Recreational activities enjoyed
  - Leisure time activities pursued
  - Sports enjoyed as a participant or observer
- Living arrangements:
  - Alone, with family members, or with others
  - Number of rooms
  - Number and ages of other individuals in home
  - Feelings about home arrangements
- Significant stressors
- Coping ability
- <u>Feelings about self:</u> Self-concept, functional status, adaptations, independence, body image, marital status, sexuality, sexual orientation
- <u>History of interpersonal trauma:</u> Rape, incest, abuse as child or spouse, other personal tragedies. Note ability to discuss, current stage in resolution (denial, fear, anger, adaptation), and resources.
- Periods of grief and current status
- Understanding of and feelings about current illness(es)
- Feelings about retirement (past, present, or future)
- Psychological problems and conflicts
- Feelings about past, present, or future caregiver roles (care for children, disabled adults, older family members)
- Spiritual concerns and needs:
  - Concept of God
  - Source of strength

- Value placed on religious practices and rituals
- Perceived relationship between religious beliefs and client's current state of health
- Spiritual adviser
- Role and relationship with an organized religious group

MENTAL STATUS ASSESSMENT
Children and Adolescents

Specific components of the mental status assessment are appropriate for most all clients beginning at about age 2. Assessment of the child will include interviews with the parents about the child as well as with the child, developmental assessment, and the physical and neurologic assessments. Direct observation of the child in a familiar environment, often during play, is also important. See Johnson and Baggett (1995, pp 17–20) for information about specific mental health interview and assessment guides for children and adolescents.

Adults

Mental status assessment is often neglected in the process of health assessment, especially in an acute care setting when physical signs and symptoms predominate. However, it should not be neglected because many mental health problems go undetected and eventually cause severe consequences for clients and their families. A baseline mental status assessment should be made on admission to a hospital or long-term-care facility. Clients who are acutely ill often manifest changes in mental status. For example, an older client hospitalized for major surgery or other illness may be confused or disoriented because of *delirium* (a temporary, usually reversible, condition caused by a physical factor such as medication), but the health-care provider may assume the confusion is caused by *dementia* associated with aging (an example of ageism or myth about the aging process). Gallo et al. (1995) stress that "the discovery of cognitive impairment should prompt a search for an etiology" (p 12). For example,

31

memory loss may be a symptom of depression rather than dementia. The nurse should assess, record, and report *any* changes in mental or cognitive status so that a specific diagnosis can be made and treatment started.

Assessing orientation to person, place, and time (often the *only* portion of the mental status examination made) may not be accurate or helpful in some situations. Knowledge of exact place or time may not be possible or important to some residents of long-term-care facilities because they do not have access to clocks, calendars, or daily newspapers. On the other hand, some clients may be able to state person, place, and time correctly but be unable to write an organized sentence or copy a simple diagram (Gallo, 1995, p 36). Therefore a more thorough assessment should be made.

General Components of the Mental Status Assessment

- Level of consciousness
- <u>Appearance:</u> Dress, hygiene, grooming, mannerisms, gestures
- Eye contact
- Position, posture, gait
- Orientation:
    - <u>Person:</u> First and last name
    - <u>Place:</u> Name of facility or home address
    - <u>Time:</u> Year, month, date of month, day of week, season, a.m. or p.m.
- <u>Speech:</u> Volume, clarity, speed, quantity, tone, accent
- <u>Language:</u> Fluency, comprehension, word choice, native language
- <u>Affect:</u> Alert, calm, responsive
- <u>Mood:</u> Feelings such as sad, depressed, joyful
- <u>Memory:</u> Immediate, recent, remote, old

- <u>Intelligence:</u> Mental development, thinking skills, vocabulary, calculation
- <u>Abstract thinking:</u> Judgment, proverbs, analogies
- <u>Attention span:</u> Intense, distracted, severely limited
- <u>Thought content:</u> Depression, paranoid beliefs, obsessions, hallucinations, phobias, delusions, illusions
- <u>Thought process:</u> Logical, spontaneous, flight of ideas, bizarre, tangential
- <u>Writing:</u> Ability to write a sentence or copy a figure
- <u>Insight:</u> Awareness and meaning of illness
- <u>Attitude:</u> Cooperative, evasive, passive, hostile
- <u>Activity level:</u> Appropriate, restless, lethargic
- <u>Response to assessment:</u> Cooperative, quiet, argumentative

Note

See the Sample Mental Status Assessment Flow Sheet (Hogstel, 1991) in Appendix D and the Mini-Mental State Examination (Folstein, Folstein, and McHugh, 1975) in Appendix E. Numerous other standardized tools to assess mental status may be found in Gallo et al. (1995). Several of these are short and rather simple to use.

FUNCTIONAL ASSESSMENT

Functional assessment is an essential component of the total health assessment. Some questions to be answered include:

- Is the person functioning at the appropriate developmental level based on age and other characteristics?

- If not, exactly which functions are not being performed? What are the reasons for the lack of or difficulty in functioning?

- What is the individual client's, family's, and healthcare provider's perception or report of level of functioning? Sometimes clients report a <u>higher</u> level of functioning than do either family members or nurses (Gallo, Reichel, and Andersen, 1995). Older people particularly may rate their health as good when their health is poor based on objective data (Sidell, 1999).

- What is the degree or level of functioning for each ability?
  - Completely independent (needs no assistance)
  - Minimal assistance needed to perform
  - Maximum assistance needed to perform
  - Completely dependent (needs total assistance)

- What assistance does the client need to be able to function as normally as possible in society? (For example, some clients need wheelchairs for mobility although they live alone and function well.)

- Where should the client and family be referred to obtain the necessary assistance to maximize the client's potential despite handicaps that limit functioning?

Functions to be Assessed (Adults)
Physical Activities of Daily Living (PADL)

- Eating
- Bathing
- Dressing
- Grooming

- Toileting
- Transfer
- Walking

Instrumental Activities of Daily Living (IADL)

- Housekeeping
- Using the telephone
- Managing money
- Preparing meals
- Driving
- Shopping
- Traveling
- Taking medications correctly
- Taking out the garbage

It is difficult to assess level of many of these functions in an acute care or clinical setting, especially at a time when the person is least likely to be functioning at a normal level because of the effects of an acute medical condition, surgery, anesthesia, and medications. Therefore, reports of the client and family may be used. However, observation of the performance of these functions will probably be more accurate than reports by clients or family members (Gallo, Reichel, and Andersen, 1995, p 72). Home-health-care nurses and nurses in other community settings are more likely to make accurate assessments of ongoing functional status. It is especially important for nurses to obtain an initial assessment of functional status on admission to home-health-care services, community clinics, and long-term-care facilities so that status over time can be evaluated.

Functional Assessment Tests

There are numerous functional assessment tests that have been developed and used extensively.

Newborns

- Apgar (see App. G): This is a functional assessment test administered to newborns to assess physiologic adaptation in the first minutes of life.

Infants and Children

- Denver II Test. This screening tool evaluates functional status in the areas of personal-social, language, fine motor, and gross motor skills in children up to age 6.

Adults

- Katz Index of Activities of Daily Living (see App. F): This is a widely used scale that assesses bathing, dressing, toileting, transfer, continence, and feeding on three levels: independent, assisted, and dependent (Katz, Ford, and Moskowitz, 1963).

- Barthel Index. This scale helps determine whether people are able to care for themselves and has been used to document improvement (Mahoney and Barthel, 1965).

Many health institutions and organizations have developed their own functional assessment tools, and in fact, qualification for covered health services (e.g., home health care under Medicaid) may depend on level of functional status in some states.

REVIEW OF SYSTEMS (SYMPTOMS)

The review of systems (sometimes called the *review of symptoms*) helps the nurse to focus on each major system of the body, noting from the health history which systems may have special problems. This systematic process prevents the omission of important assessment information.

See Part 3, "Body Organ and System Assessment," for specific questions to ask about each system.

- General
- Integument (skin, hair, nails)
- Head
- Eyes
- Ears
- Nose and sinuses
- Mouth and throat
- Neck
- Lungs and thorax
- Breasts and axillae
- Cardiovascular system
- Abdomen
- Musculoskeletal system
- Male genitourinary system and rectum
- Female genitourinary system and rectum
- Neurologic
- Adaptations in pregnancy

PEDIATRIC ADDITIONS TO THE HEALTH HISTORY

Personal Data

- Child's nickname
- Parents' telephone numbers (home and work)
- Legal agreements affecting custody

Reason for Seeking Health Care (Chief Complaint)

- Person who wanted the child to see a health-care provider (child, parent, teacher)

History of Previous Illness

- Parents' reaction to child's illness

37

- Child's response to previous treatment or hospitalization

PAST HEALTH HISTORY
Mother's Health during Pregnancy

- Age
- <u>Any drugs taken:</u> Prescription, nonprescription, alcohol, illegal drugs
- Whether pregnancy was planned
- Complications
- Illnesses
- Concerns
- <u>Exposure to toxins or other hazards:</u> Radon, chemicals

Natal and Childhood History

- Length of gestation
- Location of birth
- <u>Type of labor:</u> Induced, spontaneous; <12 hours, >24 hours
- <u>Delivery:</u> Spontaneous, forceps, cesarean; anesthesia
- <u>Apgar scores:</u> See Appendix G.
- Birth weight
- Complications

Neonatal History

- Congenital anomalies
- Condition of infant
- Oxygen and/or ventilator use
- Estimation of gestational age
- <u>Problems:</u> Feeding, jaundice, respiratory distress
- Age at discharge from hospital

- Weight at discharge from hospital
- <u>First month of life:</u> Family adaptations, responses to baby, perceived ability of family to care for baby

Infant and Childhood History

- <u>Illnesses:</u> Note exposure, specific disorders, residual effects.
- <u>Allergies:</u> Note eczema, allergic rhinitis, hives, vomiting after introduction of new foods, diarrhea.
- <u>Immunizations:</u> Note each vaccine, age when received, reactions. See Appendix H for immunization schedule.
- <u>Screening tests:</u> Note types and the child's age when each test was performed (vision, hearing, scoliosis, sickle cell anemia, tuberculosis, lead).
- <u>Operations and/or hospitalizations:</u> Note the child's and parents' reactions to the events.
- <u>Accident and/or trauma history:</u> Note consistency of explanations and emotional response to questioning if abuse is suspected.

Feeding History

- <u>Feedings and/or supplements:</u> Type, amount
- Weight gain
- Age at which solid foods were started
- Type of solid foods fed
- Infant's responses to foods
- Parents' responses to feeding their infant
- Weaning
- Food preferences
- <u>Current feeding:</u> Type, schedules
- Ability to feed self

Developmental History (See also App. I)

Note the child's height and weight at different ages, as well as the age when the child was able to:

- Hold head up
- Roll over
- Reach for toys
- Sit alone
- Crawl
- Stand alone
- Walk
- Say first word
- Talk in two-word sentences
- Dress self
- Use the toilet (urination, bowel movement)

  Sexual Development, Education, and Activity

  - Present status of sexual development
  - Age of voice change and pubic hair growth (boys)
  - Age of breast development and menarche (girls)
  - Social relations with same and opposite gender
  - Curiosity about sexuality
  - Masturbation
  - Contraception
  - Parental responses and instructions to the child about sexuality and dating
  - Child's use of language to discuss sexuality (Note age appropriateness and indicators of precocity. Note behaviors suggestive of sexual abuse.)

Social History

- <u>Sleep:</u> Patterns, problems, terrors
- <u>Speech:</u> Stuttering, delays
- <u>Habits:</u> Rocking, nail biting
- <u>Discipline used:</u> Type, frequency, effectiveness, attitudes, response of parents to temper tantrums
- <u>School:</u> Current grade, any preschool attendance, adjustments, failures, favorite subjects, performance, problems
- <u>Social behavior:</u> Relationships with peers, parents, authority figures; type of peer group, level of independence; interests and/or hobbies; self-image (If infant, toddler, or preschooler, note child-parent interactions, demonstration of affection, willingness of child to separate from parent [least likely age 8 to 20 months], evidence of increasing independence and competence.)

Family History

- Maternal gestational history
- Any consanguinity in family
- Employment history
- Child care arrangements
- Adequacy of clothing, food, transportation, sleep arrangements
- Parents' relationship with each other
- Parents' illnesses
- Siblings' relationship to one another
- Siblings' illnesses

Safety History
Infants and Small Children

- Use of infant seat or seat belts

- Placement and inaccessibility to child of poisons, household cleaning products, medications, firearms, and matches
- Presence and placement of fire extinguishers and smoke detectors
- Infants sleeping on their back or side, not abdomen
- No bottle propping
- No milk or sweetened fluids at night in crib
- Stairway gates, window guards, pool gates
- Access to syrup of ipecac, poison control center phone number
- Effect of passive smoking
- Temperature setting of hot water heater (should be ≤120)
- Use of bicycle helmet

Teens

- Assess tobacco, alcohol, and drug use.
- Assess sexual practices, risk of hepatitis B, HIV, or other STDs.
- Assess water safety practices. Remind not to swim alone or dive into water of unknown depth.

GERIATRIC ADDITIONS TO THE HEALTH HISTORY

Immunizations

- <u>Pneumonia vaccine:</u> Dates. If received before 1983, before age 65, or if person is at high risk of getting the disease and was immunized more than 5 years ago, revaccination may be necessary.
- <u>Influenza vaccine:</u> Date of last immunization. Recommended to be given annually from mid-October through mid-November.

- <u>Tetanus:</u> Date of last administration. Recommended every 10 years. If the individual never received a primary series against tetanus and diphtheria as a child, the adult should receive a series of three vaccinations (the first doses at least 4 weeks apart and the third dose 6 to 12 months later).

Current Prescription Medications

It is helpful to have the patients bring in all medications.

- Names of the medications
- Prescribing health-care professional(s)
- Prescribed dosages (assess whether the client is overdosing or underdosing)
- Side effects
- Adherence problems
- Ability to afford the medications
- Ability to get to the pharmacy
- Difficulty swallowing
- Client's opinion of efficacy of medications
- Client's use of borrowed medications
- Understanding of total medication regimen (purpose, method, timing, action, dose, side effects, interactions)
- Use of any memory aids (e.g., pill boxes, egg carton, alarm)
- Difficulty administering the medications (because of visual impairments, cognitive impairments, problems with manual dexterity)

Current OTC Medications

- Names of the medications
- <u>Dosages:</u> Amount, frequency (especially note high doses of vitamins)
- Reasons for taking

- Side or adverse effects
- Home remedies, folk medicine, herbal preparations

Nutrition

- <u>Salt and sugar intake:</u> Note whether the client adds salt or sugar to food at the table or in cooking; the amount of sugar used on cereal and in coffee and/or tea; other food items with high salt or sugar content.

- <u>Weight:</u> Note any weight changes (up or down) in the client over the past month, year, or 5 years. Client's perception of weight.

- <u>Special diet:</u> If the client follows a special diet, note the type and any difficulty adhering to the diet. Assess knowledge of diet. Does the client use any dietary supplements (kind, amount, frequency)?

- <u>Food preferences:</u> Note client's current food likes or dislikes, amounts of food consumed at one time, frequency of meals, typical meals.

- <u>Appetite:</u> Note whether the client's hunger is more pronounced at certain times of the day or night; any loss of or increase in appetite recently or over the past year; any recent changes in kinds of food eaten.

- <u>Food purchase and preparation:</u> Note who buys and prepares the food and whether the client likes it. If client prepares own food, note whether preparation is a problem. if so, is problem caused by fatigue, eating alone, decreased vision, memory impairment, or difficulty using the refrigerator or stove?

- <u>Ingestion:</u> Note any difficulty the client has in feeding self, chewing, swallowing, or choking. Are there any tooth or mouth problems? Does the client have dentures, and, if so, are they in good repair, do they fit properly, and does the client wear them? Are there certain consistencies of food the client avoids?

- Affordability: Note whether the client is able to afford the food needed and desired.

Activities of Daily Living (See also App. E)

Note whether the client requires any assistance in:

- Dressing: Fastening buttons, zippers; tying shoes
- Grooming and hygiene: Trimming fingernails or toenails, shaving, brushing teeth, brushing hair
- Bathing: Tub or shower, preparing bathwater, getting into or out of the tub or shower, washing all body parts
- Toileting: Continence, getting into the bathroom, getting onto and/or off the commode, hygiene after elimination
- Mobility: Getting into and/or out of bed, lowering into and/or getting up from chairs, transferring from bed to chair, walking, climbing stairs, reaching for items in cupboards, opening doors, recent falls
- Eating: Handling utensils, cutting food, putting food into mouth
- Laundry: By hand or with washing machine
- Meal preparation: Planning, preparing, and serving adequate meals
- Housekeeping: Making the bed, cleaning the house, washing dishes, taking out the garbage
- Financial affairs: Paying bills, balancing the checkbook
- Shopping: Transportation to store, making selections, paying for items appropriately
- Medication administration: Adhering to regimen, medication set up or assistance needed
- Transportation: Public transit, drives own car, relies on friends and/or family, public agency

Note

If the client needs assistance with any of the above activities, determine the amount of assistance needed and any adaptive equipment used. Does the client have adequate support systems available to provide the necessary assistance needed? Do family and/or friends know where and how to access the needed services?

Social Support and/or Resources (See also App. J)

- <u>Community involvement:</u> Church involvement, volunteer work, employment, hobbies, group memberships, social and/or recreational programs, classes

- <u>Support system:</u> Family and/or friends, amount of contact, type of relationship and contact, pets

- <u>Living arrangement:</u> Who lives with client and where does client live (own home, apartment, retirement community, nursing home, assisted living facility)

- <u>Finances:</u> Amount and/or source of income, type of health insurance coverage, perception of adequacy of income to meet needs

- <u>Legal services:</u> Assistance utilized. Does client have a will, a durable Power of Attorney, Medical Power of Attorney, advance directive?

- <u>Community services:</u> Does the client use such services as homemaker services, adult day care, home health care, meal assistance programs and/or nutrition sites, financial assistance programs, senior centers, home repair services, rehabilitation services?

CULTURAL AND ETHNIC ASSESSMENT

It has become increasingly important for nurses to include cultural awareness and sensitivity as essential components of the health history and physical examination processes. Demographic trends have revealed an increase in the ethnic heterogeneity of the population (see Table 3–1). These factors have greatly increased the number of clients for whom primary prevention, health education, and long-term care are important nursing interventions. If nursing interventions are to result in effective client outcomes, the nurse must understand the client's culture including lifestyles, living environment, values, and beliefs. Knowledge of the client's culture will assist the nurse in the interpretation of the client's attitudes and behaviors and facilitate the development of an appropriate health history, physical examination, and plan of care. Culture is an essential component of the knowledge base of nursing, and cultural awareness is a necessary component of nursing care.

Culture influences all learned human responses including the development of the individual's value system, behaviors, attitudes, and perceptions of the world. When values and be-

TABLE 3–1	A PROFILE OF MINORITY PERSONS AGE 65 AND OLDER IN 1998
Race and Ethnic Group	**Minority Persons Age 65 and Older = 15.7%** **(% of Minority Population)**
African American	8.0
Hispanic Origin	5.1
Asian or Pacific Islander	2.1
American Indian or Native Alaskan	<1.0

Source: Adapted from *A profile of older Americans:* 1999 Washington, DC: American Association of Retired Persons and the Administration on Aging, U.S. Department of Health and Human Services, p. 4.

liefs are culturally influenced, health and illness behaviors, communication patterns, diet, lifestyle, and religious practices also are influenced. *Clients have the right to receive care that is culturally acceptable to them.* The nurse must recognize that each person is unique and that individuals who share the same cultural or ethnic background or religious affiliation do not necessarily share values, beliefs, or cultural traditions. Nurses must assess their cultural beliefs about health and illness and avoid *ethnocentric behavior* (the belief that their own cultural beliefs and practices are superior to those of other cultures). Effective client care is enhanced in an environment that includes cultural sensitivity, mutual respect, and support and that ultimately promotes a therapeutic communication and nurse-client relationship.

An essential component of the nursing process is the observance and assessment of the client's response to perceived or actual health problems. The nurse must effectively collaborate with clients from diverse ethnic and cultural populations during cultural assessments and physical examinations to obtain accurate data that will be used to develop mutual health goals, appropriate nursing interventions, and increased client adherence. The provision of culturally sensitive care will be validated by the feedback from the client, family members, and observations of positive changes in the client's condition or behavior. Thus, the inclusion of the cultural assessment in the total client assessment is essential for providing care to a diverse population.

Cultural and Biological Traits of an Individual
Physical Appearance (Body)

- Age and developmental stage
- Gender identity
- Gender, height, weight
- Skin color

- <u>Hair:</u> color, configuration, presence or absence
- <u>Race:</u> Self-identified, perceived by others
- Posture, facial expression and variations in physical factors
- Grooming, personal hygiene
- <u>Dress:</u> Style, condition
- Presence of physical disability

Mental Characteristics and Psychological Orientation (Mind)

- Cognitive ability, intelligence
- Level of consciousness
- Emotional disposition, temperament
- Aptitude, ability
- <u>Sensory acuity:</u> Visual, auditory
- Personal traits
- Mental health status

External Influences (Social and Physical Environment)*

- Family history, ancestry, geographic origin
- Strength of family unit, lines of authority
- Role in family, birth order
- Languages, communication patterns
- Expectations and behavioral norms for age, gender, role
- <u>Format (rituals) for major life events:</u> Birth, marriage, illness, death

---

*Sources: Adapted from Geissler, E: Quick Reference to Cultural Assessment, Mosby, St Louis, 1994; and Long, BC, Phipps, WJ, and Cassmeyer, VL: Medical-Surgical Nursing: A Nursing Process Approach, ed 3. Mosby, St Louis, 1993.

- <u>Economic and work opportunities:</u> Access to resources
- Housing, living arrangements
- Dominant religion, other religions or spiritual beliefs
- Theories of disease causation
- Availability, quality, variety of health-care services
- Political, governmental structure
- Dietary customs, access to food
- Community resources in education, art, music, recreation
- Geographic and climatic features

Internal Synthesis of Body, Mind, and Environment (Self)

- Self-concept, self-perception, expectations of self
- Beliefs, values, spirituality, religious affiliation
- Affect, mood, congruity between words and affect
- <u>Personal goals:</u> Short and long term
- <u>Work role;</u> economic contribution to self, others
- Areas of accomplishment, achievement; sources of pride
- Knowledge base, utilization of educational opportunities
- Response to stress, coping strategies, ability to adapt
- <u>Language usage:</u> Formal, slang, dialect
- Food preferences, dietary restrictions
- Interests in applied and fine arts, crafts, hobbies, music, literature
- Reading ability and preference

Cultural Assessment Guide

The cultural nursing assessment is the systematic appraisal of individuals or groups about cultural beliefs, values, and practices to determine nursing needs and interventions based on cultural factors. The cultural nursing assessment provides an extended data collection tool for the recording of pertinent cultural factors that are vital to the client's acceptance and compliance to the medical regimen, nursing interventions, and behavior modification plans. The cultural aspects of the client's lifestyle, health beliefs, and health practices are essential elements that will enhance the nurse's decision making and judgment when planning and providing effective nursing care.

A thorough cultural assessment should be implemented during the initial history-taking interview with each client. (See App. K for a sample cultural assessment guide.) The cultural assessment guide will provide documentation of the information concerning the client's traditional cultural values and beliefs, communication and language patterns, and most importantly, the daily living patterns. The cultural assessment guide will also serve as a reference for other members of the health-care team when providing care. The nurse will analyze the data, formulate goals with the client when necessary, implement nursing interventions, and evaluate the goals.

The nurse should be prepared to interview the client and obtain as much information as possible concerning the client's ethnicity and dominant cultural group practices. The nurse plans for an organized sequence of data collection with specific assessment categories in which information about the client is gathered. The major categories of a comprehensive cultural assessment should include:

- Historical origin of the cultural group:
  - History and origin of ancestors
  - Length of time in original country and in current environment
- Physical presentation:

- Attire, demeanor, relationship of person(s) accompanying the client
- Communication and language patterns:
  - Literacy
  - Dominant language used in the home and understanding of the English language
  - Verbal and nonverbal messages and meanings
  - Titles, proper forms of greetings and respect
  - Improper topics of conversation
- Value and belief systems:
  - Worldview
  - Traditional values and adaptations to dominant culture norms
  - Code of conduct (ethics), behavior patterns, authority, responsibility
  - Attitudes toward time, work, play, money, education
- Religious beliefs, practices, and rituals:
  - <u>Type:</u> Traditional or modern
  - Symbols of worship, important emblems, icons
  - <u>Rituals and/or traditions:</u> Special celebrations, holidays (fertility, birth, puberty, marriage, death)
- Family roles and relationships:
  - Relative patterns
  - Marriage
  - <u>Family functions:</u> Organizations, roles, activities
  - Parenting styles
- Support systems:
  - Extended family organization and members
  - Community resources
  - Cultural group affiliations

- Social systems:
  - Economics
  - Political
  - Education
- Diet, food habits, and rituals:
  - Beliefs and significance of food
  - Adaptations when cultural food is not available
  - Rituals
- Health and illness belief systems (see App. L):
  - Values and beliefs
  - Use of nontraditional, folklore remedies and treatments
  - Acceptance and use of traditional and alternative health-care services
  - Health and/or illness behaviors and decision making

The nurse should communicate directly with the client when the individual's health condition permits. However, there are very likely to be other significant people in the client's life with whom the nurse will be required to interact when completing the cultural nursing assessment. When caring for clients from culturally diverse backgrounds, it is necessary to identify those significant others whom the client perceives to be important and who may be responsible for decision making that affects his or her health care. The nurse should be informed about the cultural values and traditions when working with a specific cultural group and enhance these cultural norms whenever possible. Consequently, supportive family members and significant others are very important factors in clients' decision making and should be included as active participants during the cultural nursing assessment.

It is also very important for the nurse to consider the fact that during the cultural nursing assessment, all historical reminiscences will not be pleasant for the culturally diverse client.

Consequently, recalling memories of traditional values, beliefs, rituals, former homelands, and family members can evoke very strong emotions for the client. The nurse should be prepared to provide the culturally appropriate support to the client. The nurse should be respectful, empathetic, supportive, facilitating, and understanding. A quiet environment that allows enough time for the client to provide the information should be maintained, and above all, good listening skills should be utilized by the nurse.

FAMILY ASSESSMENT

- Interview all family members at the same time to observe communication and decision-making patterns.
- Assess each family member's health.
- Assess family's health history:
  - Complete a genogram or family tree.
  - Include at least two generations back.
  - Include ages at death and causes of death.
  - Note patterns of illness distribution across generations (for example, cancer and heart disease).
- <u>Assess family structure:</u> Single, nuclear, nuclear dyad, extended and/or multigenerational, single parent, stepfamily, same gender.
- Assess family roles (Freidman, 1992):
  - Formal:
    - Breadwinner(s)
    - Homemaker(s)
    - Childrearer(s)
    - Financial manager(s)
    - Chauffeur(s)
    - Cook(s)
    - House repair
  - Informal roles (selected):

- Encourager (praises others)
- Harmonizer (mediator)
- Blocker (opposer)
- Compromiser (yielder, comes halfway)
- Dominator (manipulator)
- Blamer (faultfinder)
- Scapegoat (recipient of family's hostilities)
- Caregiver (nurturer)
- Assess family health:
  - Concepts of health and illness
  - Perceived level of health
  - Family health promotion strategies
  - Family stressors
  - Family strengths
  - Support systems
  - Family diet, mealtime practices, who prepares meals
  - Family activities
  - Time taken for sharing
  - Spirituality
  - Participation in the community
  - Is home a place for respite, for nurturing?
  - Health-seeking behaviors:
    - Physical examinations
    - Dental care
    - Family physician
    - Emergency department use
    - Immunization status
  - Source of insurance, adequacy of coverage
- Assess family income:
  - Source(s)

- Adequacy
- Assess family power (Friedman, 1992):
  - Assess who makes decisions about:
    - Household management
    - Discipline of children
    - Financial matters
    - Health care
    - Family leisure time activities
  - Assess who makes the decision and/or wins when major decisions are made.
  - Assess type and sources of power used by family.
  - Legitimate: One person is the authority, and this authority is believed by all family members to be appropriate.
  - Helpless and/or powerless: The victims (disabled family members or the children, for instance) gain power secondary to their helplessness.
- Referent power: Power gained from family member's positive identification (parental power).
- Resource and/or expert power: Power is based on who has the most resources (attributes, possessions, expertise). For example, family member who controls the finances may control decision making in general.
- Reward power: When one family member has the power to reward other members
- Coercive power: When power is gained through the use of violence, threats, or coercion
- Informational power: Power gained by persuasion
- Affective power: When power is gained by controlling the allocation of affection or sex
- Tension management power: When power is gained through the use of tears, disagreements, or pouting
- Assess power or decision-making process:

- **Consensus:** Mutual agreement
- **Accommodation:** Concessions made
- **De facto:** No decisions made
- Assess family communication patterns (Clark, 1999) (Fig. 3–1):
  - **Dysfunctional patterns:**
    - **The wheel:** One person directs all communication.
    - **The chain:** Communication goes "down the line" without opportunity for interaction.
    - **The isolate:** One person excluded.

The Wheel

The Chain

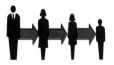

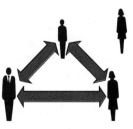

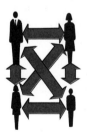

The Switchboard

The Isolate

FIGURE 3–1
Family communication patterns.

- <u>Functional pattern of communication:</u> The switchboard (communication between all members in all directions)
- Assess family developmental stage (Stanhope and Lancaster, 1996)*
  - Beginning family: Establish marriage.
  - Early childbearing family: Stabilize family, facilitate developmental needs of family members.
  - Family with preschool children: Maintain marriage, nurture and socialize children.
  - Family with school-age children: Maintain marriage, socialize children, and promote their school achievement.
  - Family with teenagers: Maintain marriage, maintain parent-child communication, build foundation for future family stages, balance teen freedom/responsibility.
  - Launching family: Readjust marriage, launch children as young adults, assist aging parents.
  - Middle-age family: Strengthen marriage, maintain relationship with children/parents, provide healthy environment, cultivate leisure activities.
  - Aging family: Adjust to retirement, reduced income, health problems, death of spouse; maintain satisfactory living arrangement.
  - Parenting practices:
    - Hopes and plans for children
    - Uses parenting styles learned from own parents
    - Disciplines children
    - Empowers children

---

*Source: Adapted from Stanhope, M, and Lancaster, J: Community Health Nursing: Promoting Health of Aggregates, Families, and Individuals, ed 4. Mosby, St Louis, 1996, p 464.

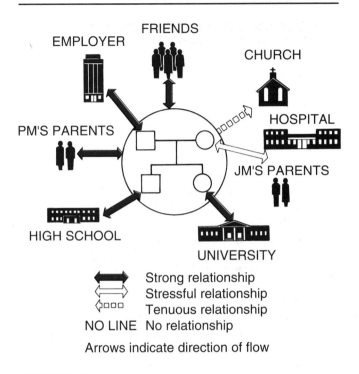

FRIENDS
EMPLOYER
CHURCH
HOSPITAL
PM'S PARENTS
JM'S PARENTS
HIGH SCHOOL
UNIVERSITY

Strong relationship
Stressful relationship
Tenuous relationship
NO LINE No relationship

Arrows indicate direction of flow

FIGURE 3–2
ECOMAP depicting family and interacting systems.

- Develops positive attitudes in children toward education, religion, athletics, extracurricular activities
- Role-models for children and teaches altruism, respect for others
- Draw ECOMAP depicting family in the center circle with spokes drawn to interacting systems. Depict direction of energy exchange and presence of stressful or tenuous relationships (see Fig. 3–2).

FAMILY CAREGIVER ASSESSMENT

When one family member is ill or disabled, another family member often takes over the role of family caregiver. In home health or hospice settings, that role often makes the difference as to whether the family member can remain at home. The nurse in those settings will need to conduct either a complete family assessment or at least the following, more focused family caregiver assessment.

Overview

- Age
- Relationship to care recipient
- Number of months since onset of caregiving
- Number of hours per day spent in caregiving
- Feelings toward caregiving: Both negative and positive, advantages, and disadvantages
- Knowledge of care recipient's care needs (physical and emotional)
- Knowledge of care recipient's medications
- Knowledge of what is involved in the care
- Evaluation of whether care recipient can be left alone
- Evaluation of what care recipient can do for himself or herself
- Evaluation of whether the care recipient's dependency has increased in the last month
- Personal medical problems
- Personal medications
- Personal illness patterns
- Personal sleep patterns:
    - Length
    - Pattern of interrupted or uninterrupted sleep
    - Place for caregiver to sleep

- Personal nutrition
- Personal exercise
- Personal stress reduction activities
- Frequency of leaving the home; purpose, duration
- Availability and use of respite services: Hospital, nursing facility, family, friends, church
- Number of times in last year care recipient has been hospitalized
- Number of times in last year care recipient was hospitalized to provide caregiver with needed rest
- Assistance caregiver identifies as being needed

If the care recipient is a client of home health care, assess if caregiver also is in need of, and potentially eligible for, home health services:

- Is the care recipient confined to the home? confined to bed?
- Does she or he need skilled care such as direct care, teaching, or monitoring of a changing condition by a registered and/or licensed nurse?
- Is she or he under the care of a physician, who would agree that home-health-care services are needed and order them?

ENVIRONMENTAL ASSESSMENT
Hospital or Nursing Facility

- Observe the client's facial expression and posture in bed.
- Note the placement and position of bed.
- Check the bed and bed rails for proper functioning and position.
- Assess any equipment attached to the client and/or bed such as nasogastric tubing, urinary catheter, IV, or monitor for proper functioning.

- Make sure that the call cord, the telephone, paper wipes, and water (if allowed) are within easy reach of the client.
- Note whether privacy and space for the client's personal possessions are adequate.
- Note any unusual odors emanating from the client or in the room.
- Note whether the floor is free from litter and moisture.
- Make sure no unnecessary equipment and/or supplies are in the room.
- Make sure lighting is adequate.

Home*

- <u>Neighborhood location:</u> Urban, suburban, rural
- Sidewalks, paved streets, presence of churches, schools, playgrounds, industries and/or businesses
- Traffic patterns in neighborhood
- <u>Size and type of home:</u> Apartment, house, trailer
- Description of home
- Whether client owns or rents the home
- Length of time in current home
- Distance to shopping
- Type of water supply
- Type of sewage disposal
- Type and efficiency of heating and cooling systems
- <u>Type of transportation:</u> Car, bus, walking

---

*Source: Adapted from Browning, M: Home environment assessment guide. In Hogstel, M (ed): Nursing Care of the Older Adult, ed 3. Delmar, Albany, NY, 1994, pp 592–595.

- Presence of a telephone or emergency signaling system
- <u>Neighbors:</u> Proximity: whether client perceives as supportive or threatening
- Adequacy of lighting outside and inside, including nightlights
- Distance to streetlights, fire hydrant, fire station
- Visibility of path from car to house by neighbors
- General cleanliness and whether home is infested with insects or rodents
- Safety of the inside and outside stairs, number of steps
- Security of the outside doors
- <u>Activities of neighborhood residents:</u> Children at play outdoors, transient persons, older residents' visibility, activity after dark
- Client's perception of safety for self in environment; client's awareness of crimes in area, perception of own vulnerability; degree to which precautions or fear affects daily activities
- Availability of safe source of heat and, if appropriate, air-conditioning
- Presence, placement, and functioning of smoke alarms
- Presence and placement of fire extinguishers
- Safety of the bathroom floor, tub, commode; functioning of the fixtures; raised toilet seat, grab bars near toilet or in tub, shower seat
- Temperature of the hot water $\leq 120°F$
- <u>Condition of the floors and stairs:</u> Cleanliness, evenness, freedom from clutter, presence of throw rugs, adequacy of lighting at night
- Width of hallways and doorways for maneuverability of walker or wheelchair

- Proximity of bathroom to bedroom
- Hospital bed located for convenience of family caregivers and for opportunity of interaction with family
- Safety and state of repair of the furniture
- Safe use of appliances and electrical cords
- Functioning refrigerator, stove
- Presence of books, radio, television, newspaper, magazines
- Proper storage of household cleaners
- Proper storage of food and medicines
- Availability of laundry facilities
- Availability and functioning of lawn equipment

SUMMARY AT END OF TOTAL HEALTH HISTORY

Ask whether there is anything else that the client would like to tell or ask you.

The Physical Examination

CHAPTER 4

PHYSICAL EXAMINATION GUIDELINES

See Appendix M for a Sample Physical Assessment Form, Appendix N for the Seven Warning Signs of Cancer, and Appendix O for a Suggested Schedule of Health Screening for People Age 65 and Older with No Symptoms.

INTRODUCTION

The physical examination generally follows the history. There are several purposes for the examination. First, baseline norms are established for the client, such as skin color and temperature and heart rate and rhythm. Second, the client's physical status is accurately described, identifying potential and actual health problems. Third, the examination allows the nurse to document history data, such as auscultating a cardiac arrhythmia after the client has described breathlessness and a fast pulse.

The physical examination is an important step in the establishment of a therapeutic relationship with the client. The client's personal needs for such things as warmth or modesty should be acknowledged and respected. The purposes of the examination are explained, and the client should be encouraged to ask questions and give responses. This is an excellent opportunity for teaching, and the examination procedures can be practiced with accompanying teaching; for example, a heart rate of 76 is normal for the client's age and activity.

PREPARATION GUIDELINES

- Provide a warm, comfortable, private environment with natural lighting, if possible.
- Eliminate distractions and disruptions.
- Check all needed equipment for proper functioning, and place it within easy reach. Explain equipment as it is used.
- Introduce yourself to the client by name and title if you have not already met the client. Unless you are in an acute care setting or an emergency, it is preferable to meet the client in a less threatening manner, for example, with the client clothed, sitting, and giving history data.
- Have the client void before the examination; collect clean specimen if needed.
- Explain each step as the examination progresses. Tell the client how much time will be involved in the entire examination. Offer general health promotion guidance with each system; for example, explain that a breast self-examination should be performed every month.
- Avoid telling jokes, inappropriate familiarity, and casual or careless touching.
- Warm your hands and instruments before touching the client's skin.

PHYSICAL EXAMINATION GUIDELINES

- If you are right-handed, stand on the client's right side. Move to the client's back (for posterior thorax) and to the client's left side (for left eye), as needed. You should be able to circle the bed or table.

- Drape the client well, exposing only those areas that are being examined.

- Be aware of your nonverbal communication during the examination; avoid frightening, intimidating, or embarrassing the client.

- Warn the client when any part of the examination may be uncomfortable.

- Be as gentle as possible.

- Be especially careful when examining sensitive areas (eyes, breasts, genitals).

- Always wear gloves when you may come in contact with body fluids or open lesions or if you have open areas in your skin.

- Carefully assess those areas where potential problems or concerns were discovered in the history and review of systems.

TECHNIQUES IN PHYSICAL ASSESSMENT
Inspection

This step is observation and visual examination. It is systematic, orderly, and purposeful, for example, examining the skin for color and hair growth patterns. Inspection requires good lighting, preferably natural daylight. The area to be inspected must be fully exposed and observable. Systematically observe color, size, shape, symmetry, and position of any lesions. See Appendix M for specific examples of each of these descriptors. Inspection may include asking the client to perform certain tasks, such as exhaling against pursed lips. Inspection may also include touch, such as squeezing the fingers and assessing blood return. Note any impairment of function.

Auscultation

This examination technique consists of listening to sounds within the body, such as the sounds of respiration or peristalsis. Most auscultation is indirect and involves the use of a stethoscope. Direct auscultation uses only the nurse's ears, and may be used to identify crepitus or an asthmatic wheeze.

The stethoscope should be no longer than 12 inches and short enough to be functional and comfortable. The flat diaphragm is used to hear higher-pitched sounds, and the bell is used to hear lower-pitched sounds:

- Use stethoscope diaphragm for bowel, breath, and cardiac sounds. Use bell for vascular and cardiac sounds.

- Assess for loudness, pitch, quality or nature, frequency, and duration (see Table 4–1).

TABLE 4–1	AUSCULTATION SOUNDS	
Type of Sound	**Description**	**Examples**
Pitch	Number of vibrations a second	Bronchial sounds ↑ Some heart sounds ↓
Intensity (strength, depth)	Soft	Normal breath sounds over lungs ↓
	Loud	Bronchial sounds over trachea ↑
Duration (length of time)	Short	Heart sounds
	Long	Bowel sounds
Quality (nature, characteristics)	Clear	Normal breath sounds
	Whistling	Abnormal breath sounds
	Musical	
	Gurgling	Stomach sounds

Source: Adapted from Kozier, B, Erb, G, Blais, K, Wilkinson, JM: Fundamentals of Nursing, ed 6. Addison-Wesley, Redwood City, CA, 1999, pp. 470–471.

Percussion (See Fig. 4-1)

In this examination technique, the examiner thumps an area of the body and observes for vibrations or sounds. Indirect percussion is the most common method, and it involves the nurse's striking a finger that is placed on the client's body part.

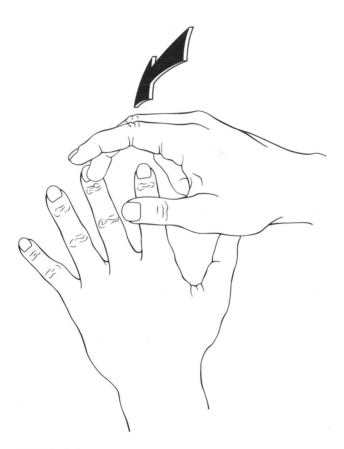

FIGURE 4-1
Percussion technique.

TABLE 4–2	PERCUSSION SOUNDS	
Tone	**Characteristics**	**Possible Source**
Tympanic	Loud, clear, drumlike	Low density, such as abdominal distention with gas
Resonant	Hollow, loud	Mixed density, such as healthy lung
Hyperresonant	Echoing, hollow	Mixed density, such as emphysematous lung
Dull	Quiet, thudding	High density, such as liver
Flat	Quiet, short, flat	High density, such as bone, thick muscle

Percussion requires knowledge of anatomic location of internal organs and their approximate size. The technique is a nonintrusive way of determining the size of organs and masses. it may also be used to estimate the tissue and contents of an organ or mass, for example, a solid mass or a bladder filled with urine.

- <u>Indirect method:</u> Place middle finger only of nondominant hand on area to be percussed. Using the tip of the middle fingernail of the dominant hand, strike the nondominant resting finger with a quick bouncing blow. Compare the sounds on the right and left sides of the area being percussed, and compare the sounds with the percussion sounds chart (see Table 4–2).

Palpation

This examination technique uses touch to gather data. The fingertips are most often used to palpate lightly, for example, to elicit incisional pain, or deeply, for example, to determine the presence of a kidney. Deep palpation is rarely indicated in general nursing practice.

Assisting the client to relax during palpation, especially when examining the abdominal area, will enhance the accuracy of the findings. Allow the client to control the timing of the palpation, and be alert to cues of discomfort.

Method

- Palpation requires touching with different parts of the hand and with varying degrees of pressure to determine characteristics of pain, temperature, size, shape, moisture, and/or texture.

- Explain reason for touch to client. Warm hands.

- Use light palpation before deep palpation.

- Use pads of fingers (most sensitive part) to identify texture, size, shape, or movement (e.g., pulse).

- Use dorsum of fingers for temperature assessment.

- Gently pinch skin to assess turgor on forehead or upper third of sternum.

- Use palms or ulnar side of hand to assess vibrations.

- Use deep palpation gently and briefly to assess areas such as pelvis and abdomen for body organs and masses.

- Palpate painful areas last.

PEDIATRIC ADAPTATIONS
General Guidelines

- If the child does not know you, it is best if there is someone else in the room whom the child trusts, preferably a parent or other family member.

- Parents can assist by telling you how they cope with the child.

Suggestions for Specific Age Groups
Younger Infants

- Let the parent assist by holding the child on his or her lap.
- Avoid chilling.

Older Infants

- Parents should be within the child's view.
- Move slowly, and approach the child slowly.
- Restrain the child adequately and gently with parents' assistance.

Toddlers and Preschoolers

- Keep the parents in the room; ask them to assist when appropriate.
- Tell the child that it is all right to cry or yell.
- Allow the child to play with the equipment if desired (during the history taking).
- Use distraction.
- Perform the least threatening parts of the examination first.
- Use a doll to demonstrate certain parts of the examination.
- Restrain the child adequately.
- Use the parents to assist (e.g., holding stethoscope on the child's chest).
- Give the child simple choices when possible.

Preschoolers

- Explain briefly what the child will experience.
- Demonstrate the equipment; allow the child to play with it or use it on a doll.

- Let the child know that the examination is not punishment.
- Involve the child by allowing him or her to hold the chart or stethoscope for you.
- Praise the child for helping and cooperating.

School-Age Children

- Explain the examination and allow time for questions.
- Explain what you are doing.
- Allow the child to assist by handing equipment to you.
- Allow the child to listen, feel, or see what you find.
- Protect the child's privacy.

Adolescents

- Explain the examination and encourage questions.
- Examine the child apart from the parents and ask if there are any questions.
- Tell the child the findings and the norms (e.g., "Your breasts are beginning to develop; that is normal for a 12-year-old").
- Protect the child's privacy.

GERIATRIC ADAPTATIONS

General Guidelines

- Prepare the environment, taking into account sensory and musculoskeletal changes:
  - Allow adequate space to accommodate mobility aids.
  - Use straight-backed chairs rather than low, soft, curved chairs.

- Minimize background noise and distraction, such as TV, radio, intercom system, or nearby communication between other people.
- Avoid glossy or highly polished surfaces (floors, walls, ceilings, or furnishings).
- Use a well-padded, low examination table.
- Maintain close proximity to restroom facilities.
- Diffuse lighting with increased illumination (avoid using direct or fluorescent lighting). Avoid having client face glare from windows.
- Ensure a comfortable, warm room temperature.
- Maintain complete privacy for client.

- Conduct the examination, taking into account the energy level, pace, and adaptability of the older adult:

  - Allow ample time for the exam because older clients may move more slowly and take longer to react and respond to questions. Be alert to signs of fatigue, and consider conducting the exam in more than one session.
  - Approach the client in a relaxed and unhurried manner.
  - Allow the client ample time to respond to questions and directions.
  - Use silence to allow the older client time to collect thoughts before responding.
  - Sit facing the client to facilitate eye contact, lip reading, and rapport (see Fig. 4–2).
  - Use commonly accepted vocabulary and clear questions or instructions.
  - A visual deficit may warrant the use of frequent verbal cues and touch.
  - A hearing deficit calls for lowering the voice pitch, speaking slowly, and avoiding shouting.

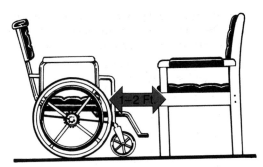

Sitting in chair or wheelchair:
  sit very close to (1–2 feet away) and
  facing the client.

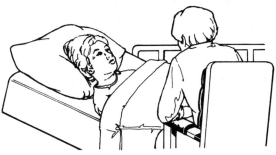

Lying in bed:
  sit level with the client, and maintain
  a close position facing the client.

FIGURE 4–2

Optimal seating positions for communication with the older adult.

You may need to resort to writing information or possibly using an amplified listening device.

* Never leave older clients unattended on an exam table, as they could fall off while adjusting their position.

* Assist the older client on and off the examination table and with position changes to avoid injuries.

* To conserve the client's energy, organize the examination to minimize position changes.

* To avoid chilling and protect modesty, keep the client warmly covered and expose only the body part being examined.

Possible Modifications

* If the client has breathing problems or a curvature of the spine, it may be necessary to elevate the examining table and/or use pillows.

* If the client has a musculoskeletal disorder and/or feels dizzy, some neurologic tests may need to be omitted.

CULTURAL AND ETHNIC VARIATIONS*

* Allow ample time for examining the ethnic client because of possible language differences, increased sensitivity with the exposure, observation, and palpation of body parts and the close proximity of the nurse to the client.

* Be aware of nonverbal communication during the examination. Avoid sudden moves, extreme facial gestures, and hurried mannerisms, all of which may heighten intimidations, embarrassment, fear, insecurity, and lack of trust about the examination.

---

*Source: Adapted from Muecke, MA: Culture and ethnicity. In Craven, RF, and Hirnle, CJ, Fundamentals of Nursing: Human Health and Function. Lippincott, New York, 1992, pp 236–252.

- If a language interpreter is necessary, speak to the client rather than to the interpreter; doing so enables the client to "read" the nurse's nonverbal language.

- Avoid using metaphors and idioms unless the nurse is knowledgeable regarding language variations.

SUGGESTED SEQUENCE OF THE PHYSICAL EXAMINATION

Note

The following sequence illustrates one method to integrate all systems for a complete examination at one time. This method focuses on efficiency of time and helps protect and preserve the client's energy. This section presents an overview of the sequence of the physical examination. Part 3 presents the details for the examination of each body system.

Examination
Overview

- Vital signs (radial pulses), blood pressure (BP)
- Height, weight
- Speech, cognition, mental status, interaction
- Gait, Romberg, coordination, balance

Integument (*Client Sitting*)

- Inspect and palpate all visible skin surfaces.
- Evaluate lesions (draw if helpful).
- Inspect hair and nails.

Head

- Inspect, palpate

- Cranium
- Eyes, cranial nerves (CN) II, III, IV, V, VI
- Ears, CN VIII
- Nose, CN I
- Sinuses
- Mouth, CN XII
- Throat, CN IX
- Preauricular and postauricular and occipital nodes

Neck

- Inspect, palpate, auscultate
- Carotid pulses
- Thyroid gland
- Lymph nodes
- Range of motion (ROM), CN XI
- Jugular veins

Back

- Inspect, percuss, palpate, auscultate
- Fremitus, respiratory excursion
- Symmetry, spinal alignment
- Costovertebral angle tenderness
- Mobility

Anterior Trunk (*Client Seated and/or Lying*)

- Inspect the breasts.
- Auscultate breath sounds, heart sounds, carotid pulses, apical impulse (compare rate of apical impulse with radial pulse).
- Assess ROM of upper extremities.
- Palpate brachial pulses.
- Palpate the breasts, axillary, and epitrochlear lymph nodes.

- Palpate thrills, point of maximum intensity.
- With client on left side or leaning forward, auscultate apex for murmurs.

Abdomen

- Inspect movement, color, contour.
- Auscultate the four quadrants.
- Auscultate for bruits over abdominal aorta, renal artery, iliac artery, and femoral artery.
- Percuss the abdomen.
- Palpate the abdomen.
- Palpate and/or percuss for bladder distention.
- Measure the size of the liver.
- Palpate the inguinal nodes, femoral pulses.
- Assess ROM of remaining joints if the client is unable to stand.
- Palpate popliteal, dorsalis pedis, and posterior tibial pulses.

Musculoskeletal System

- Assess weight bearing, gait, posture.
- Check extremities for edema.
- Inspect and palpate upper and lower extremities and joints for tenderness, heat, crepitus.
- Assess muscle development, symmetry, tone.
- Check ROM of lower extremities, equal length of extremities.

Neurologic System

- Assess color, warmth, strength, ROM, gait, gross motor movement.
- Test the reflexes: Biceps, triceps, brachioradialis, patellar, achilles, plantar.
- Test balance, proprioception, fine motor movement.

- Test the cranial nerves if not previously tested.
- Test sensory perception.

Genitourinary System (*Client Standing and in Lithotomy Position*)

- External and internal genitalia
- Pap smear
- Rectal examination
- Prostate examination

GENERAL GUIDELINES FOR DOCUMENTATION OF FINDINGS

- Documentation of assessment is an important communication step. Without adequate recording, the assessment is limited in its use and value. Documentation helps the health-care team exchange information and prevents the client from enduring needless repetitions. The client's record is a confidential, consistent source of data about the client, both baseline data and changes in condition, as well as treatments and responses.

- In addition to communication, the written medical record serves other purposes. It is a legal document, and parts of it may be admitted into evidence in court. The record can be thought of as a legal description of the client's experience with health-care providers. A common saying in clinical settings is "if it was not charted, it was not done." Without documentation in the record, for example, the nurse may have a difficult time convincing a jury that the client was assessed appropriately before the administration of a medication.

- The medical record also provides a source of data for audits, statistical analysis, and research. For example, a nursing quality management committee may review a series of records of discharged clients to determine the consistency of documentation of assessing venipuncture sites. Research may be conducted by evaluating the interventions recorded regarding cleansing urinary catheters of immobile clients. Incidences of nosocomial infections can be tracked by the infection control nurse.

- Finally, client medical records may be seen as care studies for students in the health-care field. The written chronology of a client's experience provides students with human responses to illness. For example, the medical record may illustrate the changes in laboratory data as a client with liver failure begins to decline.

- The system of documentation varies widely in agencies and institutions. The nurse may record data on a computer terminal at the bedside, write in a descriptive narrative in longhand, or use a series of abbreviations, symbols, and acronyms on a standardized flow sheet. Follow the appropriate form, and use only those abbreviations accepted by the agency or institution. If a narrative is required, record findings in a manner that is clear, concise, complete, accurate, and systematic.

- Examples of documentation can be found at the end of each body system section. The following guidelines may be useful in writing narratives:

  - Record all names, dates, and times fully and clearly on the right chart.

  - Write legibly.

  - Record statements or descriptions without bias or undue interpretation. For example, if a client accuses a nurse of following him and snooping into his affairs, the nurse should record the statements and behaviors of the client rather than describe the client as paranoid.

  - Avoid generalizations. Rather than "wound appears infected," make note of the color, swelling, temperature, drainage, and presence of pain.

- Always document exceptions, abnormalities, or changes in the client's condition. For example, any arrhythmia, bleeding, or cyanosis should be reported and documented.

- Note normal findings in situations when abnormalities might be expected. For example, a pregnant woman with hypertension, visual disturbances, and epigastric pain could be expected to demonstrate hyperactive deep tendon reflexes. Therefore, even if the reflexes are a normal +2, this information has particular significance.

- Record changes in behavior or physical condition, especially noting full date and exact time. If the sclera are slightly jaundiced, for example, documentation and reporting of this change, as well as noting its previous absence, will facilitate the medical response.

- Document as quickly as possible after the action, sign all notes, and avoid recording for others except in unusual circumstances. Keep notes until you chart them.

- In case of late additions to charting or an error, follow agency or institution policy, noting exact date and time.

Suggestions for Ease in Recording

- Record findings on the form provided by the institution (if available).

- If the institution does not have a specific form for documenting assessment data, use the nurses' notes to record the assessment, following a systematic approach (based on a specific order of systems and a specific order within each system).

- Document (record) all normal and abnormal physical findings in a clear, organized, readable, succinct, systematic manner.

- Use only abbreviations and terms accepted by the institution or agency.

- Use a capital letter at the beginning and a period at the end of each statement. Use other punctuation as needed for clarity. Complete sentences are not necessary.

- Some institutions have bedside computer terminals so that assessment data can be recorded in the client's room as soon as possible. Written data can usually be added to the hard copy.

REMEMBER

For diagnostic, treatment, and legal reasons, it is better to record too much than too little.

Body Organ and System Assessment

CHAPTER 5
GENERAL OVERVIEW (WITH EXAMPLES)

Note and Document the Following Information about the Client:

- <u>Apparent age:</u> Compared with stated or actual age.
- <u>Weight:</u> Note if clothing and/or shoes are included in measurements.
- <u>Height:</u> Remove the client's shoes.
- <u>Arm span:</u> Equal to height except in older clients because of decreasing height with increasing age.
- <u>Vital signs:</u> Take blood pressure (BP) in lying, sitting, and standing positions. Repeat in other arm if elevated. Do not take BP in arm on mastectomy side or limb with dialysis access.
- <u>Body type:</u> Tall, short, obese, thin, unusual body build.
- <u>Posture:</u> Straight, stooped.
- <u>Gait:</u> Fast, slow, limping, shuffling.
- <u>Body movements:</u> Mannerisms, tremors.
- <u>Obvious odors:</u> Alcohol, perfume, infection, poor hygiene.
- <u>Personal hygiene:</u> Hair, oral hygiene, nails.

- <u>Manner of dress:</u> Style, casual, hospital gown.

- <u>Speech:</u> Clear, weak, slurred, hesitant, stuttering.

- <u>Affect:</u> Flat, hostile, alert.

- <u>Mood and manner:</u> Cheerful, depressed, crying.

VITAL SIGNS

Equipment

- Thermometer, lubricant, watch with second hand, stethoscope, sphygmomanometer, gloves, disposable sheaths

Assessment of the Adult

Health History

- Inquire about known temperature elevations, elevated blood pressure, pulse, and breathing problems.

Temperature

- Inquire about recent ingestion of fluids, food, or smoking within last 10 minutes.

- Secure appropriate thermometer, and shake down to 94°F (34.4°C) if mercury-in-glass type is used. Apply disposable sheath if applicable.

- <u>Oral:</u> Place tip of thermometer near base of tongue; close lips. Keep in place 3 minutes if using mercury-in-glass thermometer or until beeps are completed if using electronic thermometer. Normal range is 97.5 to 99.5°F (36 to 38°C).

- <u>Rectal:</u> With client in left lateral Sims' position, gently insert lubricated tip 1 to 1.5 in. Hold in place 3 minutes if using mercury-in-glass thermometer or until beeps are completed if using electronic thermometer. Normal range is 98 to 100.5°F (37 to 38.8°C)—usually 0.5 to 1°F higher than oral.

- <u>Axillary:</u> With client's arm raised, place tip of thermometer at center of axilla. Lower arm completely. Leave in place 7 to 10 minutes. Normal range is 96.5 to 99°F (35 to 36.8°C). Axillary: Usually 0.5 to 1°F lower than oral.

- <u>Tympanic membrane:</u> Place clean disposable cover on the ear speculum. Gently pull pinnae back. Insert speculum gently into external ear canal. Thermometer registers in seconds. Normal range is approximately the same as the oral method, 97 to 100°F (36 to 37.8°C).

Pulse

- <u>Rate:</u> Palpate radial pulse for 30 seconds and multiply times 2. Count for 1 full minute if irregular. Also assess for regular rhythm, strength (full, not bounding or thready), and equality (compare left and right). Normal range is 60 to 100 beats per minute.

Respiration

- <u>Rate:</u> Count breaths for 1 minute; normal range is 12 to 20 per minute. Also assess depth and rhythm and use of accessory muscles.

Blood Pressure

- Auscultate BP in sitting position with brachial artery at level of heart. Auscultate in standing and lying positions. Assess lying BP first if assessing for postural hypotension. Repeat in other arm if elevated. Do not use the arm on the side of a mastectomy or dialysis access. Normal ranges:

  - <u>Systolic:</u> 96 to 140 mm Hg
  - <u>Diastolic:</u> 60 to 90 mm Hg

- Blood pressure should not drop 20 mm Hg or more as the client rises from a sitting to a standing position.

Pediatric Adaptations
Temperature

- <u>Rectal:</u> Place child prone on bed or across parent's lap. Use one arm across buttocks to restrain. Insert lubricated thermometer 0.5 to 1.0 in. Hand holding the thermometer should be braced against child's body to prevent injury.

- <u>Tympanic membrane:</u> Use ear tug to ensure accuracy. Pull pinnae down and back. Explain device before approaching child, who may perceive the apparatus as a gun.

- <u>Ranges:</u>

<u>Age</u>	<u>°C</u>	<u>°F</u>
Newborn to age 1	37.7–37.5	99.7–99.4
ages 3–5	37.2–37.0	99.0–98.6
ages 7–9	36.8–36.7	98.3–98.1
age 10 and older	36.6	97.8

Pulse

- Use apical rate, not radial.
- <u>Ranges of heart rates:</u>

Newborn	80–160
1 week to 3 months	80–180
3 months to 2 years	80–150
2 years to 10 years	70–110
10 years to adult	55–90

Respiration

- Most accurate rate is counted when child is sleeping. Watch movement of the abdomen of infant.

- <u>Ranges of respiratory rates:</u>

Newborn	30–40
1 year	20–40
2 years	20–30
5 years	20–25
10 years	17–22
15 years	15–20

Blood Pressure

- <u>Ranges:</u>

Age	Systolic/Diastolic (mm Hg)
1 month	86/54
1 year	96/65
4 years	99/65
6 years	100/60
8 years	105/60
10 years	110/60
12 years	115/60
14 years	118/60
16 years	120/65

Geriatric Adaptations*

Temperature

- Tympanic membrane thermometer is ideal because it is quick and safe.

- Oral method may not be accurate if the person cannot keep the mouth closed for the required length of time.

- Rectal or axillary methods should not be used unless absolutely necessary.

- Note that older adults may remain afebrile during an infection because of a lower baseline temperature and a decreased immune response.

Pulse Rate

- No major changes in old age but may decrease in persons age 85 and older.

Respiration

- Depth may decrease and rate may increase.

---

*Source: Adapted from Hogstel, MO: Vital signs are really <u>vital</u> in the old-old. Geriatric Nurs 15(5):252–256, 1994.

| TABLE 5-1 | VITAL SIGNS FOR PERSONS 85 OR OLDER COMPARED WITH YOUNGER ADULTS |

	Age Group	
Vital Signs	**Adults Aged ≥18***	**85 and Over**
Temperature (°F):		
Oral	98.6°	95–97° (average 96.8°)
Tympanic membrane	97.6°	94–96°
Axillary	97.8°	94–96°
Rectal	98.8–100.2°	95.2–98.6°
Pulse rate (beats per minute)	70 (male) 75 (female)	70–75 (no major change; resting pulse may be lower)
Respiration (breaths per minute)	15–20	20–22 (more shallow)
Blood pressure (mm Hg)	120/80	<140/90†
Pulse pressure (mm Hg)	30–50	50–100‡

*Traditional norms are given for the adult age 18 and over for comparison purposes, although it is recognized that there are ranges of norms for individuals depending on time of day, activities, sex, weight, diet, and emotions.
†Systolic and diastolic may increase, but that is not normal.
‡Pulse pressure may widen in the absence of disease.
Data for this table were compiled from the following sources:
Britten, MX: Assessing and maintaining body temperature. In Sorensen, KC, and Luckmann, J (eds): Basic Nursing, ed 2. WB Saunders, Philadelphia, 1986, p 556.
Kozier, B, Erb, G, and Olivieri, R: Fundamentals of Nursing, ed 4. Addison-Wesley, Menlo Park, CA, 1991, pp 324–525, 667.
Potter, PA, and Perry, A: Fundamentals of Nursing, ed 3. Mosby–Year Book, St Louis, 1993, pp 461, 469.
Source: Hogstel, MO: Vital signs are really *vital* in the old-old. Geriatric Nurs 15(5):254, 1994, with permission.

TABLE 5–2	ETHNIC VARIATIONS IN VITAL SIGNS			
Group	**Temperature (°F)**	**Pulse**	**Respiration**	**Blood Pressure**
African Americans	97.8°	84	18	130/86
Asian Americans	97.0°	72	14	110/66
Native Americans	99.8°	90	20	136/88
Hispanic	98.8°	84	16	130/80

Sources:
Cox, CR, and Bloch, B: Sociocultural and spiritual dimensions of health. In Berger, KJ, and Williams, MB (eds), Fundamentals of Nursing Collaborating for Optimal Health. Appleton and Lange, East Norwalk, CT, 1992.
Muecke, MA: Culture and ethnicity. In Craven, RF, and Hirnle, CJ, Fundamentals of Nursing: Human Health and Function. Lippincott, New York, 1992.
Seidel, HM, Ball, JW, Dains, JE, and Benedict, GW: Mosby's Guide to Physical Examination, ed 4. Mosby, St Louis, 1999.

- If you experience difficulty counting, observe and count the rise and fall of the abdomen.

Blood Pressure

- Normal systolic and diastolic BP are the same as in other adults. Pulse pressure (systolic-diastolic) may increase.

See Table 5–1 for normal ranges in persons age 85 and older.

RACIAL AND ETHNIC VARIATIONS

See Table 5–2 for ethnic variations in vital signs.

CHAPTER 6
INTEGUMENT

HISTORY

> ### Note
> A brief review of the essential components of the history is included at the beginning of each system. In many clinical situations the nurse will be concentrating primarily on one or more systems rather than a total integrated health assessment.

Adult

- Past skin diseases
- Years of exposure to sun, use of tanning beds, and other environmental factors
- Recent change in a wart or mole (see App. P)
- Any sore that has not healed
- Rashes, lesions, abrasions, bruises
- Tick bites
- Adverse effects of medications
- Allergies, seasonal or climatic effects
- Recent changes in hair growth, distribution
- Recent changes in nails (e.g., ridges, thickening, color bands)
- Recent changes in sensation of pain, heat, cold
- Thyroid, endocrine, and circulatory disorders

Pediatric
Infants
- Type of diaper and diaper cream used
- Method and products used for bath
- Rashes, lesions, bruises
- Injuries

Pediatric
Children
- Injury history related to play (e.g., abrasions, cuts)
- Signs of abuse
- Allergies
- Acne, eczema; include onset, treatment
- Recent exposure to a communicable disease

Geriatric
- History of skin cancers or other chronic skin conditions
- Excessive dryness, itching
- Increased bruising tendency
- Increased healing time
- Chronic long-time sun exposure
- Marks (excoriation, redness, trauma)
- Temperature changes in skin
- Nail texture changes
- Frequency of bathing and products used for bathing

Racial and Ethnic
- Use of home remedies or local applications of any kind on skin

- Occupational hazards (e.g., skin contact materials, radiation, abnormal lighting)

- Care of pimples or minor lesions (squeezing or picking)

- Care of excess hair (shaving, plucking)

- Excessive dryness, itching

- Use of lotions, creams, oils, and other skin lubricants

- Use of special hair products

- Use of bleaching creams and other skin-lightening or tanning agents

- Increased bruising tendency

- Increased healing time

EQUIPMENT

- 6-in transparent ruler measured in centimeters as well as inches (Fig. 6–1)

- Penlight or flashlight

- Gloves

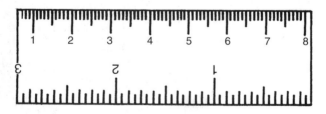

FIGURE 6–1

A ruler measured in centimeters as well as inches. A usable 6-in ruler is shown on the inside back cover of this book and a 15-cm ruler on the inside front cover.

CLIENT PREPARATION

- Have client sit and stand for total exposure of skin.

- Keep client warm.

- Maintain complete privacy.

PHYSICAL ASSESSMENT: SKIN
Adult

A

Steps	Normal and/or Common Findings	Significant Deviations
Inspection		
• *Color:* Note symmetry, shade.	Pink, light brown, dark brown, ruddy, coffee, chloasma, vitiligo	Pale, cyanotic, jaundiced, sallow
• *Lesions:* Note size, location, shape, color.	Nevi, scars, keloids, especially in dark pigmented skin (Fig. 6–2), striae	Tracks, varicosities, tick bites (whitened center with red circle around it)
• *Erythema:* Note location, size, blanching.	None	
• *Lesions:* Note type, morphology, location, size, shape, grouping or arrangement, exudate.	Macules	Papule, nodule, tumor, wheal, vesicle, bulla, pustule, erosion, excoriation, fissure, ulcer, scale, petechia, purpura, ecchymosis (Table 6–1)
Smell		
• Odors	Cigarette smoke, perspiration	Alcohol, acetone, foul odors

Table continued on following page

A PHYSICAL ASSESSMENT: SKIN *(Continued)*
Adult

Steps	Normal and/or Common Findings	Significant Deviations
Palpation		
• Temperature	Warm, cool	Hot, cold
• Turgor for degree (Figs. 6–3 and 6–4)	Rebounds instantly	Tented for >5 seconds
• Degree of moisture	Dry	Damp, clammy
• Texture	Smooth, even	Rough
• Lesions or lumps for pain, depth, size if not visible	None	Pain

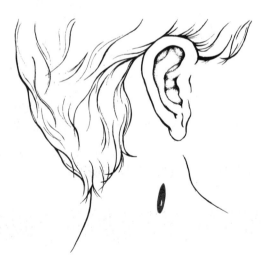

FIGURE 6–2

Keloid lesion on neck: nodular, firm area of hyperplastic scar tissue from previous surgery and/or trauma.

TABLE 6-1	TYPES OF SKIN LESIONS

Lesion	Size (cm)	Description
	PRIMARY LESIONS	
Macule	<1	Flat, circumscribed, varied in color
Papule	<1	Elevated, firm, solid
Nodule	1<2	Elevated, firm, solid
Tumor	>2	Elevated, firm, solid
Wheal	Varied	Transient, irregular, edematous
Vesicle	<1	Elevated, serous fluid filled
Bulla	>1	Elevated, serous fluid filled
Pustule	Varied	Elevated, purulent fluid filled
	SECONDARY LESIONS	
Erosion	Varied	Moist epidermal depression; follows rupture of vesicle, bulla
Excoriation	Varied	Crusted epidermal abrasion
Fissure	Varied	Red, linear dermal break
Ulcer	Varied	Red dermal depression; exudate
Scale	Varied	Flaky, irregular, white to silver
Petechia	<0.5	Flat, red to purple
Purpura	>0.5	Flat, red to purple
Ecchymosis	Varied	Dark red to dark blue, painful

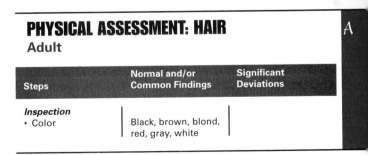

PHYSICAL ASSESSMENT: HAIR
Adult

A

Steps	Normal and/or Common Findings	Significant Deviations
Inspection • Color	Black, brown, blond, red, gray, white	

Table continued on following page

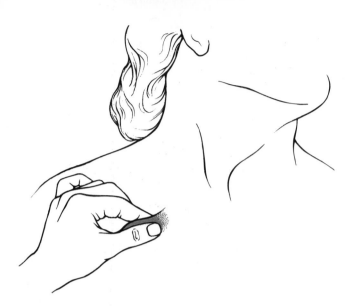

FIGURE 6–3
Testing skin turgor: adult.

PHYSICAL ASSESSMENT: HAIR *(Continued)*
Adult

Steps	Normal and/or Common Findings	Significant Deviations
• Quantity	Thick, thin, sparse	Patchy, none
• Distribution for presence, symmetry of body hair	Varies	Alopecia, marginal alopecia, hirsutism, absence on lower limbs
• General condition	Combed, clean	Dirty, uncombed, matted
Palpation		
• Texture	Coarse, fine, curly, oily, dry	Brittle

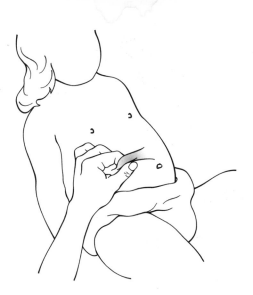

FIGURE 6–4
Testing skin turgor: child.

PHYSICAL ASSESSMENT: NAILS
Adult

A

Steps	Normal and/or Common Findings	Significant Deviations
Inspection		
• Plate for color	Pink, light brown	Blue, black
• Cuticle	Smooth	Edema, erythema, exudate
• Shape	Curved	Clubbed, flattened (see also Fig. 13–1)
• Configuration (Fig. 6–5)	Longitudinal ridges	Transverse depressions or ridges, pits
• General condition	Clean, neat	Unkempt, dirty
Palpation		
• Consistency	Firm	Boggy, brittle

SPOON NAIL (KOILONYCHIA)

SPLINTER HEMORRHAGES

ONYCHOLYSIS

PARONYCHIA

TRANSVERSE GROOVING
(BEAU'S LINES)

FIGURE 6–5

Abnormal nail conditions.

PHYSICAL ASSESSMENT: SKIN

Pediatric Adaptations
  Infant

Steps	Normal and/or Common Findings	Significant Deviations
Inspection • Color	Usually reflects a lighter shade of parents' skin color at birth; reddened to pink, acrocyanosis,* mongolian spots, harlequin sign, stork bite, mottling*	Pallor, physiologic jaundice, nevus flammeus, cyanosis, purpura, multiple bruises, lesions that may be inconsistent with history

PHYSICAL ASSESSMENT: SKIN *(Continued)*
Pediatric Adaptations
Infant

Steps	Normal and/or Common Findings	Significant Deviations
• Texture	Smooth, soft; vernix in creases if term*	Peeling
• Lesions	Milia; forceps marks on head*	Capillary hemangioma, erythema toxicum, blisters
• Integrity	Intact	Openings, clefts especially on spine, head
• Palmar, sole creases for number, pattern	Multiple creases at term	Few to absent creases; simian line
Palpation		
• Turgor on abdomen	Instant recoil	Tenting
• Lesions for size, shape, consistency		Café au lait spots > 5 mm
		Pitting edema or periorbital edema

PHYSICAL ASSESSMENT: HAIR
Pediatric Adaptations
Infant

Steps	Normal and/or Common Findings	Significant Deviations
Inspection		
• General condition	Clean; cradle cap, lanugo*	Bald spot on back of head
		Hair tuft on spine.

*Newborn only.

PHYSICAL ASSESSMENT: NAILS
Pediatric Adaptations
  Infant

Steps	Normal and/or Common Findings	Significant Deviations
Inspection • Size • Shape • Color	Thin; may be long; easily cyanotic to pink	Clubbing

 PHYSICAL ASSESSMENT: SKIN
Pediatric Adaptations
  Child

Steps	Normal and/or Common Findings	Significant Deviations
Inspection • Color	Yellowish cast from eating yellow vegetables	Multiple bruises, burns; ashen gray in dark-skinned persons
• Common diseases	Ringworm, impetigo, scabies	Varicella, candidiasis

 PHYSICAL ASSESSMENT: HAIR
Pediatric Adaptations
  Child

Steps	Normal and/or Common Findings	Significant Deviations
Inspection • Foreign bodies	Color may darken and thicken	Head lice, nits, ticks, alopecia, pubic hair on child <age 9

PHYSICAL ASSESSMENT: SKIN
Pediatric Adaptations
Adolescent

Steps	Normal and/or Common Findings	Significant Deviations
Inspection • Sebaceous glands	Oily, acne, comedones	Pitting, scarring

PHYSICAL ASSESSMENT: HAIR
Pediatric Adaptations
Adolescent

Steps	Normal and/or Common Findings	Significant Deviations
• *Body hair:* Note amount, pattern, texture.	Increases in amount; coarseness; progresses toward adult fullness and texture	Sparse, scanty, fine, patchy

PHYSICAL ASSESSMENT: SKIN
Geriatric Adaptations

Steps	Normal and/or Common Findings	Significant Deviations
Inspection • Color	*Lentigo senilis:* Back of hands, arms, face	Erythema; **bruises** (**head and trunk** more significant than arms or legs as possible signs of abuse)

Table continued on following page

103

G
PHYSICAL ASSESSMENT: SKIN (Continued)
Geriatric Adaptations

Steps	Normal and/or Common Findings	Significant Deviations
• Temperature	Cool	Uneven, asymmetrical, very cold
• Moisture	Dry, scaling, decreased perspiration	Cracked, fissured, marked flaking
• Texture	Thinning, transparent	
• *Turgor:* Check on forehead, chest or abdomen (see Fig. 6–3)	Wrinkling, decreased subcutaneous fat, sagging	Extended tenting, excessive sagging (weight loss)
• Lesions (Fig. 6–6)	Cherry angiomas, seborrheic keratosis, acrochordons, senile purpura	Actinic keratosis, basal cell carcinoma, squamous cell carcinoma, herpes zoster, pressure ulcers (Fig. 6–7 and Table 6–2)

G
PHYSICAL ASSESSMENT: HAIR
Geriatric Adaptations

Steps	Normal and/or Common Findings	Significant Deviations
Inspection		
• Color	Loss of pigment > age 50	
• Quantity	Decreased body hair, hirsutism, decreased hair on lower extremities, thinning of hair on head	Unusual alopecia, asymmetrical

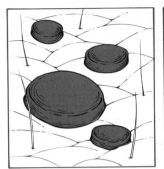

A, CHERRY ANGIOMA.

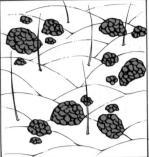

B, ACTINIC KERATOSIS.

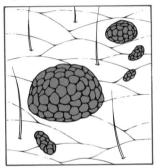

C, SEBORRHEIC KERATOSIS.

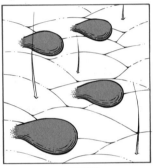

D, ACROCHORDON.

FIGURE 6–6

Common skin changes in older adults. (*A*) Cherry angioma. (*B*) Actinic or senile keratosis. (*C*) Seborrheic keratosis. (*D*) Acrochordon.

PHYSICAL ASSESSMENT: NAILS
Geriatric Adaptations

G

Steps	Normal and/or Common Findings	Significant Deviations
Inspection • Texture	Ridges, longitudinal splitting, thickening, decreased growth	

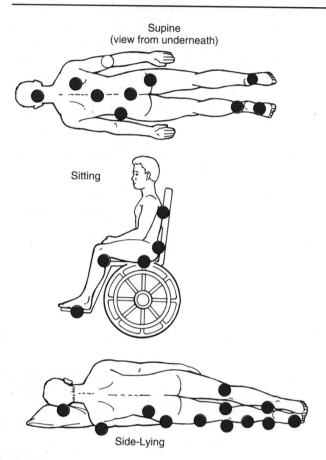

FIGURE 6–7

Body prominences prone to pressure ulcers.

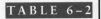

| TABLE 6-2 | **STAGES OF PRESSURE ULCERS** |

The National Pressure Ulcer Advisory Panel has classified pressure ulcers into four stages:

Stage I	Nonblanchable erythema of intact skin.
Stage II	Partial-thickness skin loss involving the epidermis or dermis.
Stage III	Full-thickness skin loss involving subcutaneous tissue that may extend to, but not through, the underlying fascia.
Stage IV	Deeper, full-thickness lesions extending into muscle or bone.
Eschar	Ulcers covered by eschar (hard necrotic tissue) are unstageable and usually represent ulcers of at least a stage III.

Source: Clinical Practice Guideline: Treatment of Pressure Ulcers. US Department of Health and Human Services, Public Health Service, Agency for Health Care Policy and Research, Rockville, Md, December 1994, vol 15.

PHYSICAL ASSESSMENT: SKIN
Racial and Ethnic Adaptations

Steps	Normal and/or Common Findings	Significant Deviations
Inspection • *Color:* Changes best observed in sclera, conjunctivae, oral mucosa, tongue, lips, nail beds, palms, soles. (Table 6–3.)	Ranges from deep black to light brown to olive and yellow overtones. Wrinkled skin areas (appear darker knees, elbows). Calloused areas appear yellow (palms, soles).	Edema causes dark skin to appear lighter. *Pallor:* Brown skin becomes yellow; black skin becomes ashen gray. Cyanosis noted in nail beds, conjunctivae, palms, soles.

Table continued on following page

R

PHYSICAL ASSESSMENT: SKIN (Continued)
Racial and Ethnic Adaptations

Steps	Normal and/or Common Findings	Significant Deviations
	Dark-skinned clients may have lips with blue hue.	Petechiae noted in conjunctivae and oral mucosa.
	Oral mucosa darker pigmentation in gums, cheeks, borders of tongue.	Signs of sickle cell disease: Jaundice, pallor, chronic leg ulcers
	Keloid scar formation after surgery, tattoos, and cosmetic piercing.	
Palpation	Smooth	Rashes may not be detected by inspection.
	Cool	Erythema not easily detected by inspection.

TABLE 6–3	ASSESSMENT OF SKIN COLOR	
Characteristic	**White or Light-Skinned Person**	**Dark-Skinned Person**
	PALLOR	
Vasoconstriction present	Skin takes on white hue, which is color of collagen fibers in subcutaneous connective tissue.	Skin loses underlying red tones. Brown-skinned person appears yellow-brown. Black-skinned person appears ashen gray.

TABLE 6-3	ASSESSMENT OF SKIN COLOR *continued*	
Characteristic	**White or Light-Skinned Person**	**Dark-Skinned Person**
PALLOR		
		Mucous membranes, lips, nailbeds pale or gray.
ERYTHEMA, INFLAMMATION		
Cutaneous vasodilation	Skin is red.	Palpate for increased warmth of skin, edema, tightness, or induration of skin. Streaking and redness difficult to assess.
CYANOSIS		
Hypoxia of tissues	Bluish tinges of skin, especially in earlobes, as well as in lips, oral mucosa, and nail beds.	Lips, tongue, conjunctivae, palms, soles of feet are pale or ashen gray.
		Apply light pressure to create pallor; in cyanosis tissue color returns slowly by spreading from periphery to the center.

Table continued on following page

TABLE 6-3 **ASSESSMENT OF SKIN COLOR** *continued*

Characteristic	White or Light-Skinned Person	Dark-Skinned Person
	ECCHYMOSIS	
Deoxygenated blood seeps from broken blood vessel into subcutaneous tissue.	Skin changes color from purple-blue to yellow-green to yellow.	Oral mucous membrane or conjunctivae will show color changes from purple-blue to yellow-green to yellow. Obtain history of trauma and discomfort. Note swelling and induration.
	PETECHIAE	
Intradermal or submucosal bleeding.	Round, pinpoint purplish-red spots are present on skin.	Oral mucosa or conjunctivae show purplish-red spots if person has black skin.
	JAUNDICE	
Accumulated bilirubin in tissues	Yellow color in skin, mucous membranes, and sclera of eyes. Light-colored stools and dark urine often occur.	Sclera of eyes, oral mucous membranes, palms of hand, and soles of feet have yellow discoloration.

Source: Adapted from Murray, RB, and Zentner, JP: Nursing Assessment and Health Promotion Strategies through the Life Span, ed 6. Appleton and Lange, East Norwalk, CT, 1997, p 47, with permission.

PHYSICAL ASSESSMENT: HAIR

Racial and Ethnic Adaptations

Steps	Normal and/or Common Findings	Significant Deviations
Inspection		
• Color	Wide variation from light brown to deep black	
• Quantity	Thick, thin, sparse	Thinning Alopecia
• Distribution	Present on scalp, lower face, nares, ears, axillae, anterior chest around nipples, arms, legs, back of hands and feet, back, buttocks	
• Texture	*Scalp:* Fine or coarse *Body:* Fine *Pubic and axillary:* Coarse	Brittle
• Lesions	Small, inflamed pustules near hair follicles	Scars or burns from heat or chemicals

PHYSICAL ASSESSMENT: NAILS

Racial and Ethnic Adaptations

Steps	Normal and/or Common Findings	Significant Deviations
Inspection		
• Color	Pigment deposits in nail beds in dark-skinned clients	

DIAGNOSTIC TESTS

- Refer to physician for biopsy of suspicious lesions.

POSSIBLE NURSING DIAGNOSES

- Infection, risk for
- Injury, risk for
- Tissue integrity, impaired
- Trauma, risk for
- Skin integrity, impaired
- Skin integrity, risk for impaired
- Self-care deficit, feeding, bathing/hygiene, dressing/grooming, toileting
- Body image disturbance
- Self-esteem disturbance
- Unilateral neglect

Clinical Alert

- Report all suspicious lesions.
- Report suspicious bruising, especially around the mouth, eyes, or ears or on the chest (could be signs of abuse).
- Note problems with cleanliness, grooming.

SAMPLE DOCUMENTATION

Skin bilaterally pale pink and elastic, with no varicosities, ecchymoses, edema, or erythema. Multiple striae present along lower abdomen and medial aspects of breasts. Abundant maculae scattered across nose, cheeks, and backs of ears. Raised white scar, 2 cm in diameter, on upper outer aspect of left arm.

Skin on extremities symmetrical, cool, and dry. No noticeable odors. Hair thick, fine, light brown, and distributed normally on head. No hirsutism or hair loss noted. Nails slightly curved, firm, with no ridges or pits. Nail beds pink. No clubbing.

CLIENT AND FAMILY EDUCATION AND HOME HEALTH NOTES

Adult

- Avoid exposure to sun as much as possible, especially between 10 A.M. and 2 P.M.
- Use sunscreens above Skin Protection Factor (SPF) 15 when possible (dark and very dark skins may use an SPF as low as 4 or 6).
- Prevent clothing from irritating moles, warts, and other lesions.
- Do total self-assessment of skin monthly.
- Do not push cuticle back from nail surface.

Pediatric
Infant

- Teach parents to avoid sun exposure for infants before 6 months of age, after which a sunscreen of 15 SPF or greater should be used.
- Teach parents about general and individual variations of normal.
- Lower water heater thermometer to 110°F.
- Test bathwater temperature before placing baby in bath.
- Instruct parents in cleansing and care of skin; use mild soap, rinse well, use oil only if very dry, and do not use powders. Wash scalp and fontanels.
- Clip nails when infant is asleep or quiet.

N

- Change diapers frequently.
- When changing diapers, cleanse from pubis to anus.

Adolescent

- Wash face with nondeodorant soap and water 2 to 3 times daily if skin is oily.
- Do not pick acne pustules.
- Continue to stress use of sunscreens.

C

Geriatric

- Use soap sparingly and rinse well.
- Avoid using harsh deodorant or perfumed soaps
- Bathe 5 to 7 times a week using tepid water rather than hot water.
- Do not use alcohol or powder on skin.
- Apply a lanolin-containing emollient after bathing (while skin is still moist) to help retain moisture absorbed while bathing.
- Avoid bath oils because they can increase the risk of falls in the tub.
- Use room humidifiers or place pitcher of water over heaters to increase moisture in the air.
- Avoid wearing rough fabrics next to the skin. Wear cotton underpants.
- Keep feet and areas between toes clean and dry.
- Use manicure stick rather than metal file to clean nails.
- Diabetics must be very meticulous with foot care (inspecting feet daily, performing foot care very carefully, and having toenails cut and/or cleaned by health professional).
- Clients restricted to bed must be repositioned frequently (at least every 2 hours). Position changes

need not be drastic; a slight change is often adequate. Bony prominences must be well padded.

- Clients restricted to wheelchair must shift their position every 15 to 30 minutes.

- Incontinent clients must practice meticulous skin care, changing absorbent product as soon as soiled, cleansing skin well after each incontinent episode, making use of moisture barrier creams, using only absorbent pads at night to allow air to reach skin, and using external collection devices.

- Refer client to podiatrist if unable to safely trim and clean toenails.

- Prevent prolonged pressure to any area by frequent position changes (every 2 hours may not be enough in high-risk patients) and range-of-motion exercises.

Other

- Teach safe use of hair care products. Comb hair immediately when wet with large-toothed comb to prevent breakage. If scalp oils are used, encourage client to read label for presence of irritants. Explain risks of hot-comb alopecia and irreversible damage (burns, scars) to scalp because of excessive heat.

- Pseudofolliculitis can occur from shaving curly, coarse hair. Discuss options such as growing a beard or using depilatory instead of razor.

- Avoid direct sun exposure if the client is using skin-lightening creams (many products have sunscreen added).

- Use sunscreen and tanning products cautiously (Jarvis, 2000).

- Sole surfaces and heels may be very calloused and cracked because of increased dry skin layers, failure to properly wash and/or clean (scraping with dull instruments or using pumice bars), improper shoe fit, and walking without shoes. Refer client to podiatrist if you are unable to safely clean or if you observe signs of irritation or infection.

- Diabetic clients should be referred to podiatrist if they have foot injuries or if they are unable to safely trim and clean toenails.

- Constricting garments (girdles, knee-high stockings, garter belts) must not be worn by clients with circulatory, endocrine, and cardiovascular problems.

- In some cultures, women do not shave body hair.

Associated Community Agencies

- Adult Protective Services (APS)
- American Academy of Dermatology
- American Cancer Society
- Skin Cancer Foundation
- National Pediculosis Association

CHAPTER 7

HEAD

HISTORY

Adult

- Risk of head injury from accidents involving automobiles, cycling, sports, job, other
- Use of helmet and seat belts
- History of head injury, seizures, headaches, dizziness

- **Headache:** Location, onset, duration, character of pain, precipitating factors, associated symptoms, treatment
- Stress management techniques

Pediatric

- Birth trauma, difficult delivery
- Neural tube defects
- Injuries (trauma, risk factors)
- Reaching developmental milestones

Geriatric

- Syncope, headaches, trauma
- Dizziness related to sudden movements of head or neck

EQUIPMENT

- Tape measure
- Pin or cotton ball
- Flashlight or penlight
- Stethoscope

CLIENT PREPARATION

- Sitting

A **PHYSICAL ASSESSMENT**
Adult

Steps	Normal and/or Common Findings	Significant Deviations
Inspection		
• *Head:* Note position, movements, facial features, symmetry, shape, expressions.	Upright Still	Tilted to one side; involuntary movements Tremor, bobbing, nodding Tics, spasms
	Slight asymmetry	Asymmetry: Entire side, partial, mouth only
	Uniform	Edema, unusual shapes
	Appropriate	Flat, fixed
Palpation		
• *Skull:* Note shape, symmetry.	Smooth, uniform, intact	Lump, indentations
• *Temporal arteries:* Note course.	Smooth, nontender	Tenderness, thickening
• *Temporomandibular joint:* Note range of motion.	3–6 cm vertical range when mouth open; 1–2 cm lateral motion; snaps or pops	Pain Crepitus Inability to close or open fully
Test		
• *Cranial nerve (CN) VII:* Have client puff cheeks, raise brows, frown, smile, show teeth.	Symmetrical movement	Asymmetrical motion or absence of motion
• *CN V:* Have client clench teeth. Touch pin or cotton ball to chin, then cheek.	Symmetrical movement Symmetrical response	Asymmetrical motion or absence of motion Asymmetrical or absent perception of touch

PHYSICAL ASSESSMENT *(Continued)*
Adult

A

Steps	Normal and/or Common Findings	Significant Deviations
Auscultation (Only if vascular anomaly suspected; use bell only.) • Temples, eyes, suboccipital areas, forehead.		Bruits

PHYSICAL ASSESSMENT
Pediatric Adaptations
Infants

P

Steps	Normal and/or Common Findings	Significant Deviations
Inspection • *Skull:* Note size, shape, symmetry (Fig. 7–1).	Molding Caput succeda- neum, flat fontanels, long narrow shape if premature	Frontal bossing Cephalohematoma Dilated scalp veins Separated sutures Flattened occiput may result from pro- longed supine posi- tioning
Palpation • *Fontanels:* Note size, tension, su- ture lines. (Hold child upright.) Posterior closes by 2 months. An- terior closes be- tween 9 and 18 months.	<5 cm anterior, slight pulsation, soft fontanel	Marked pulsations or depressed fontanels; bulging, full fontanels Nonpalpable su- tures Extra ridges, cran- iotabes

Table continued on following page

PHYSICAL ASSESSMENT

Pediatric Adaptations
  Infants

Steps	Normal and/or Common Findings	Significant Deviations
Measure • Frontal occipital circumference (FOC)	Should approximate chest circumference	Micro/macrocephaly
Transilluminate (Only if abnormality is suspected)	Light does not penetrate skull	Light glows through cranial cavity

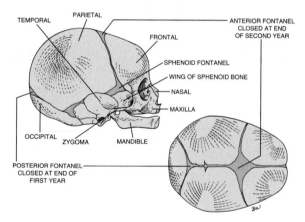

FONTANELS OF INFANT'S SKULL AND BONES OF SKULL

FIGURE 7–1

Fontanels of an infant's skull and bones of the skull. (*Source:* Thomas, C (ed): Taber's Cyclopedic Medical Dictionary, ed 18, FA Davis, Philadelphia, 1997, p 743, with permission.)

120

PHYSICAL ASSESSMENT

Pediatric Adaptations

Children

Steps	Normal and/or Common Findings	Significant Deviations
Auscultation • Eyes, temples, subocciput	Bruits common until age 4	Bruits after age 4

PHYSICAL ASSESSMENT

Geriatric Adaptations

None.

PHYSICAL ASSESSMENT

Racial and Ethnic Adaptations

Steps	Normal and/or Common Findings	Significant Deviations
Inspection • Bones	Frontal bone thicker and parietal occiput not as thick in African-American males as in white males	

DIAGNOSTIC TESTS

May need to refer for:

- CT scan
- MRI

121

POSSIBLE NURSING DIAGNOSES

- Trauma, risk for
- Tissue perfusion, altered, cerebral
- Injury, risk for
- Body image disturbance

Clinical Alert

- **Pediatric**
  - **Cephalohematoma**
  - **Bulging or depressed fontanels**
  - **Microcephaly**
  - **Macrocephaly**
- **Adult, Geriatric**
  - **Bruits**
  - **Asymmetry if marked or new**
  - **Hardness, thickening, or tenderness over temporal arteries, which may be associated with temporal arteritis**
  - **Enlarged occipital, preauricular, or postauricular lymph nodes**

SAMPLE DOCUMENTATION

Face symmetrical without involuntary movements. CN V, VII intact. Skull smooth, symmetrical. Expressions appropriate to setting. Scalp without lesions or flaking. Temporal arteries without thickness or tenderness.

CLIENT AND FAMILY EDUCATION AND HOME HEALTH NOTES

Adult

- Always use helmet when cycling.
- Always use seat belts.
- Practice basic stress management techniques.
- Do not ride or carry passenger in back of pickup trucks.
- Do not drive while under the influence of alcohol or drugs.
- Do not dive into water of unknown depth.

Pediatric

- Explain various skull shapes due to birth procedures, and indicate expected recovery time.
- Explain fontanels, including that they can be touched, and that hair should be washed.
- Strongly encourage the use of helmets when riding bicycle or skateboarding and the use of car seats and seat belts (mandatory in most states).
- Encourage parents to place infant in prone position while awake to decrease flattening of head.
- Place infant in supine or side-lying position for sleep.

Geriatric

- Provide tips related to dizziness.
- Caution client to avoid falls. Do not use throw rugs. Use safety grips on floor of bathtub, label stairs well, and use night light in bathroom.
- Rise from lying or sitting positions to standing position slowly if dizziness occurs.
- Use cane or walker if indicated.

Other

- Clients with circulatory, endocrine, and/or cardio-vascular problems should seek immediate medical attention with sudden onset of severe headaches, dizziness, blurred vision, change in level of consciousness, change in speech pattern, or irregular heart rates (high incidence and mortality rates for myocardial infarction, hypertensive crisis, and stroke).

Associated Community Agencies

- National Head Injury Foundation
- Alzheimer's Association (support services, information)
- Mental Health Association

CHAPTER 8

NECK

HISTORY

Adult

- Recent weight changes
- Changes in activity tolerance; fatigue, irritability
- Thyroid disease or surgery
- Neck stiffness, pain, and limited motion
- Temperature intolerance
- Difficulty swallowing
- Enlarged lymph nodes
- Radiation exposure
- Chemotherapy
- HIV exposure
- IV drug use

124

- Recurrent infections
- Hoarseness
- Athletic injuries to neck
- Engages in heavy lifting
- Tobacco use
- Bleeding

Pediatric
Infant

- Maternal hyperthyroidism
- Quality of head control

Geriatric

- Thyroid disease, especially hypothyroidism
- Stiff neck muscles

EQUIPMENT

- Stethoscope
- Cup of water (thyroid)

CLIENT PREPARATION

- Client should be sitting.
- Client may need a cup of water to swallow during thyroid palpation.

A

PHYSICAL ASSESSMENT
Adult

Steps	Normal and/or Common Findings	Significant Deviations
Inspection		
• *Neck:* Note shape, symmetry, size.	Uniform, symmetrical, proportional to head and shoulders	Masses, webbing, or fullness Unusually short Edema
• *Trachea:* Note position.	Midline	Deviations to either side
• Carotid, jugular	Mild pulsations	Distention, fullness
• *Thyroid (with and without swallowing):* Note symmetry, size.	Usually not visible	Marked
Palpation		
• *Trachea:* Note position, margins, motion. (Finger and thumb held on either side of trachea; feel for downward pull that is synchronous with pulse).	Midline, nontender, distinct rings	Edematous, deviated laterally, tender or painful, tracheal tugging
• *Thyroid:* Note size, shape, consistency, tenderness. Place two fingers on each side of trachea below cricoid cartilage. Feel for isthmus while client swallows. Gently	May be non-palpable. Right lobe may be slightly larger if palpable with swallowing.	Enlarged, tender, nodules, masses, roughened surface Fixed

PHYSICAL ASSESSMENT *(Continued)*
Adult

Steps	Normal and/or Common Findings	Significant Deviations
push trachea to right side, have client tilt head to left side, and feel right lobe while client swallows. Reverse and repeat. Palpate lateral borders by pressing on either side of each sternocleidomastoid as client swallows (Figs. 8–1 and 8–2).		
• *Lymph nodes:* Note location, mobility, size, shape, consistency, tenderness, skin margins, color. (Begin with light pressure, gradually increasing to moderate pressure.) See Figure 8–3 for nodes to palpate.	Nonpalpable; small (≤1 cm), smooth, firm, mobile, nontender, discrete margins	Inflamed nodes: Enlarged, tender, mobile, blurred borders, reddened skin Malignant nodes: Enlarged, nontender, fixed, hard, nodular, irregular shape, nondiscrete margins
Testing • *CN XI:* Have client shrug shoulders with and without resistance, and have client turn head to each side against resistance.	Symmetrical movement and strength	Asymmetrical or absent motion

Table continued on following page

127

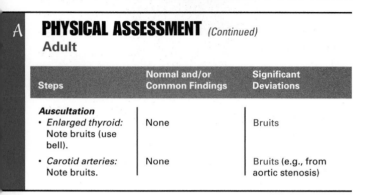

A PHYSICAL ASSESSMENT *(Continued)*
Adult

Steps	Normal and/or Common Findings	Significant Deviations
Auscultation		
• *Enlarged thyroid:* Note bruits (use bell).	None	Bruits
• *Carotid arteries:* Note bruits.	None	Bruits (e.g., from aortic stenosis)

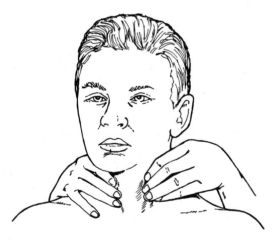

Palpating thyroid

FIGURE 8–1
Palpating the thyroid.

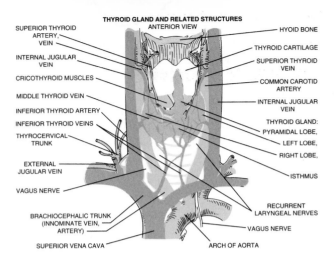

FIGURE 8–2

Thyroid gland and related structures. (*Source:* Taber's, ed 18, 1997, p 1952, with permission.)

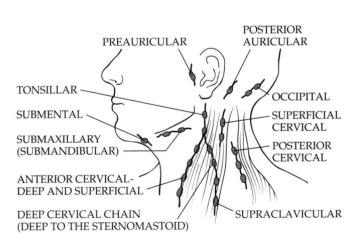

FIGURE 8–3

Lymph nodes of the head and neck.

P

PHYSICAL ASSESSMENT
Pediatric Adaptations

Steps	Normal and/or Common Findings	Significant Deviations
Inspection • Assess ROM of neck. Note nuchal rigidity, if any.	Full ROM	Webbing Nuchal rigidity Edema Head lag past 6 months Head tilt Torticollis
Palpation • Thyroid	May not be palpable, nontender	
• *> 2 years:* Postauricular and occipital. *> 1 year:* Cervical, submandibular	Lymph nodes may be palpable Midline, no deviations	
• Trachea		

G

PHYSICAL ASSESSMENT
Geriatric Adaptations

Steps	Normal and/or Common Findings	Significant Deviations
Inspection • *ROM:* Note flexibility, strength. Do ROM very slowly and carefully.	Decreased	Marked limitation of movement Crepitation back of neck (cervical arthritis)

PHYSICAL ASSESSMENT *(Continued)*
Geriatric Adaptations

Steps	Normal and/or Common Findings	Significant Deviations
Palpation		
• Thyroid	Small, smooth, or nonpalpable	Pain, dizziness
		Enlarged lobes
• Lymph nodes	May be irregular or fibrous nodules	palpable without swallowing, tenderness
Auscultation		
• Carotid arteries		Bruits

DIAGNOSTIC TESTS

May need to refer for:

- Infant screen, hypothyroidism
- Biopsy of enlarged lymph nodes
- Thyroid-stimulating hormone (TSH), triiodothyronine (T_3), thyroxine (T_4), (T_7)
- Carotid Doppler study

POSSIBLE NURSING DIAGNOSES

- Airway clearance, ineffective
- Activity intolerance, risk for
- Swallowing, impaired
- Aspiration, risk for

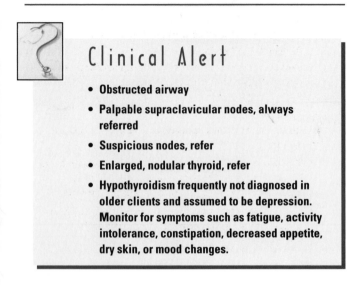

Clinical Alert

- Obstructed airway
- Palpable supraclavicular nodes, always referred
- Suspicious nodes, refer
- Enlarged, nodular thyroid, refer
- Hypothyroidism frequently not diagnosed in older clients and assumed to be depression. Monitor for symptoms such as fatigue, activity intolerance, constipation, decreased appetite, dry skin, or mood changes.

SAMPLE DOCUMENTATION

Neck smooth, supple, with full ROM. Trachea aligned in midline. No jugular venous distention. Thyroid not visible, not palpable. No tenderness. CN XI intact. Lymph nodes (auricular, occipital, clavicular, cervical, tonsillar, submaxillary, submental) not palpable. No carotid bruits bilaterally.

CLIENT AND FAMILY EDUCATION AND HOME HEALTH NOTES

Adult
- Self-referral of enlarged suspicious nodes, difficulty swallowing

Pediatric
- <u>Infants:</u> Thoroughly clean skin folds in neck.

- **Infants:** No pillows or soft stuffed animals should be allowed in crib.
- Never shake infant or child (significant risk for injury of head or neck).

Geriatric

- Refer client for thyroid tests if he or she reports low energy.
- Exercise neck muscles to maintain as much mobility as possible (flexion, extension, hyperextension, rotation, and lateral flexion).
- If several pillows are used, place part of pillows under shoulder to prevent prolonged extreme neck flexion.

CHAPTER 9

EYES

HISTORY

Adult

- Date and source of last eye exam; age at time of exam
- Use of corrective lenses; if so, type, how long
- History (self or family) of hypertension, diabetes, allergies, thyroid disorder, glaucoma, medications, color blindness
- History of previous eye surgery, trauma, infection
- Employment: risk of injury
- Participation in athletic activities, use of protective devices

133

- Headache
- Pain, burning, itching, drying, tearing, discharge
- Blurred vision
- Lights, spots, floaters
- Recent changes in vision
- Allergies

Pediatric

- Preterm: resuscitated, oxygen therapy
- Maternal rubella while pregnant
- Ability to follow object and fixate with eyes
- Squinting to see objects; rubbing of eyes
- Age, date, and source of last eye exam; age at time of exam
- Headaches when reading
- Reversals of written numbers and/or letters
- Trouble reading correctly
- Sitting close to the television at home
- Excessive tearing

Geriatric

- History of glaucoma, diabetes, cataracts, or macular degeneration
- Decreased vision, difficulty reading or seeing at night
- Peripheral or central vision blurred
- History of glaucoma in family; any acute eye pain
- Long, excessive exposure to sunlight
- Bothered by glaring lights
- Bothered by rainbows around lights or halos around lights

- Difficulty distinguishing colors
- Dry eyes
- Increased eye tearing
- Double vision, tunnel vision, or transient blindness
- Use of corrective lenses; used for what purpose?
- Use of any aids (magnifier) or any environmental adaptations to see better
- History of floaters (spots) and flashes of light

Other
- Retinoblastoma, cancer of retina
- History of strabismus
- Nocturnal eye pain

EQUIPMENT
- Penlight
- Rosenbaum chart (Fig. 9–1) or newsprint
- Snellen chart*
- Ophthalmoscope
- Clean cotton wisp
- Cover card

CLIENT PREPARATION
- Client should be in a sitting position.
- Explain darkening of room for ophthalmic exam.
- Explain use of cotton to elicit blink.

---

*Use Snellen chart (see Fig. 9–7) for children 3–7 years old.

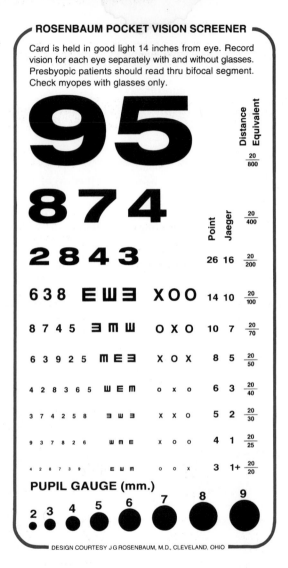

FIGURE 9–1

Rosenbaum pocket vision screener. (*Source:* Dr. J. George Rosenbaum, FACS, Cleveland, Ohio, with permission.)

136

PHYSICAL ASSESSMENT: EXTERNAL EYES

Adult

Steps	Normal and/or Common Findings	Significant Deviations
Inspection		
• Bony orbit, brows, lacrimal apparatus, eye: Note symmetry, size, position (Fig. 9–2).	Equal size and movement	Exophthalmos Strabismus
• Lids: Note position, motion, symmetry, lesions.	Symmetrical blink; lashes even and curl out, moist Xanthelasma	Edema, ptosis, exudate, ectropion, hordeolum
• Iris: Note color, shape.	Uniform color, round	Coloboma, iridectomy
• Cornea, lens (with oblique light)	Clear, smooth, moist	Opaque, arcus senilis before age 40
• Note cloudiness of lens.		Cataract
• Pupil: Note shape, symmetry, response to light.	PERRLA: Pupils equal, regular, react to light and accommodation Consensual	Not equal in shape; response to light unequal, slow, absent, diminished

Table continued on following page

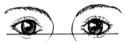

COMMON EYES

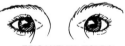

EPICANTHAL FOLDS

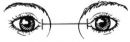

WIDE SET EYES

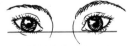

PALPEBRAL SLANT

FIGURE 9–2
Placement of eyes.

137

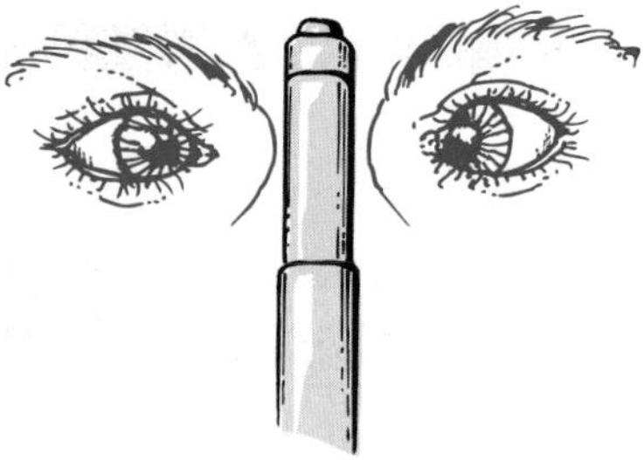

FIGURE 9–3
Checking for optical
accommodation and
convergence.

A PHYSICAL ASSESSMENT: EXTERNAL EYES

(Continued)

Adult

Steps	Normal and/or Common Findings	Significant Deviations
• *Pupil:* Note accommodation. Focus distant object, then close (Fig. 9–3).	Constricts for close object, convergence present	Miosis, mydriasis Fails to respond to focus change
• *Conjunctivae:* Note color, continuity, vascularity.	Clear with multiple small vessels	Reddened, exudate, lesions, jaundice
Palpation		
• Bony orbit	Firm, nontender	Tenderness
• Lacrimal apparatus	Pink, moist puncta	Tenderness, drainage, reddened, edema
Testing Eye Function		
• *CN II:* Rosenbaum chart at 14 in (see Fig. 9–1). Have client cover one eye, test uncovered eye.	20/20 without straining *Near vision:* Reads at 14 in	Decreased acuity, e.g., 20/40 Moves closer or further than 14 in for reading

PHYSICAL ASSESSMENT: EXTERNAL EYES

A

(Continued)
Adult

Steps	Normal and/or Common Findings	Significant Deviations
Test with lenses if client already uses glasses or contacts. Test OD, OS, OU.		
• *Confrontation test:* With your eyes level with client's eyes, stand 2 ft from client and cover one eye while client covers opposite eye. Look at each other. Move object into superior, inferior, nasal, and temporal fields for each eye (Fig. 9–4).	Object seen by both at same time	Diminished peripheral vision
• *CN III, IV, VI, and extraocular muscles:* Hold client's chin, have client focus eyes on pencil held at comfortable distance from eyes; instruct client to follow pencil with eyes as pencil is moved through six cardinal fields of gaze (Fig. 9–5).	Smooth, equal movements	Nystagmus Lid lag
• Shine light obliquely into each pupil.	Equal pupillary constriction	Asymmetry or absence of pupillary constriction

Table continued on page 141

139

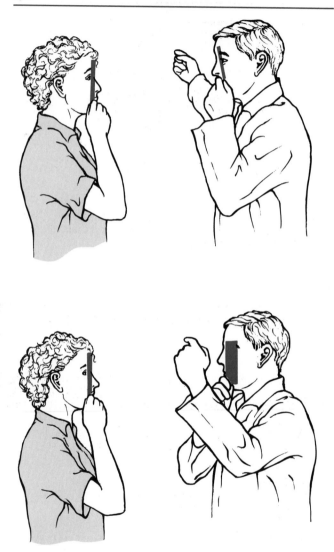

FIGURE 9–4
Testing peripheral fields of vision.

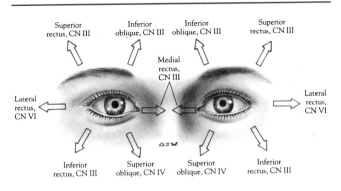

FIGURE 9–5

Extraocular eye muscles (EOM). (*Source:* Seidel, H, Ball, J, Dains, J, and Benedict, GW: Mosby's Guide to Physical Examination, ed 4. Mosby, St. Louis, 1999, p 286, with permission.)

PHYSICAL ASSESSMENT: EXTERNAL EYES

(Continued)
Adult

Steps	Normal and/or Common Findings	Significant Deviations
• Muscle balance with corneal light reflex. Shine light on corneas while client looks straight ahead.	Symmetrical reflection of light	Asymmetry; strabismus, hypertelorism
• *CN V:* Touch wisp of cotton to cornea to elicit blink reflex (alert client before touching with cotton).	Blink symmetrical and complete	Asymmetrical, incomplete, or absent blink response

A

A

PHYSICAL ASSESSMENT: INTERNAL EYES
Adult

Darken room. Have client focus on object over your shoulder. OD:
ophthalmoscope in right hand, focus with numbered wheel. OS:
ophthalmoscope in left hand. (Procedure is tiring for client.)

Steps	Normal and/or Common Findings	Significant Deviations
Inspection		
• Red reflex	Present Round, reddish orange	Cataract; hemorrhage may appear solid or as dots
• *Retina:* Note color.	Yellowish pink, uniform	Marked dark colors, lesions, folds in retina
• *Disk:* Note color, size, shape, margins of disk, and cup.	Yellow to pink, round, 1.5 mm, sharply defined border, cup 40%–50% of disk, lighter color in center of disk	Papilledema, cupping with white color, vessels visible in disk
• *Vessels:* Note color, size, junctions.	Size A3:V5, arterioles bright red	Cup less or more than 40%–50% of disk
• *Macula densa and fovea centralis:* Note location, color (Fig. 9–6). Difficult to locate unless pupils are dilated.	Located two disk diameters temporal to disk, bright yellow	Arteriovenous (AV) nicking, areas of constriction

FIGURE 9–6
Retina of right eye.
(*Source:* Taber's, ed 18,
1997, p 1670, with
permission.)

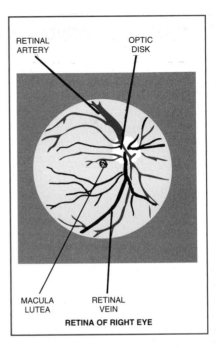

RETINAL ARTERY

OPTIC DISK

MACULA LUTEA

RETINAL VEIN

RETINA OF RIGHT EYE

PHYSICAL ASSESSMENT: EXTERNAL AND INTERNAL EYES

Pediatric Adaptations
Infant and Child

Steps	Normal and/or Common Findings	Significant Deviations
Inspection • *External eye:* Note spacing, symmetry (see Fig. 9–2).	Symmetrically positioned and spaced	Sunken eyes Edema of lids, epicanthal folds (abnormal except in Asians), hypertelorism

Table continued on following page

P

PHYSICAL ASSESSMENT: EXTERNAL AND INTERNAL EYES *(Continued)*

Pediatric Adaptations
Infant and Child

Steps	Normal and/or Common Findings	Significant Deviations
• Ability of infant to gaze at parent and blink appropriately.		Failure to gaze and blink Setting sun sign
• *Conjunctivae:* Note color, clarity.	Pink, moist	Drainage Excessive tearing Pallor
• Muscle balance	Symmetrical movement, pseudostrabismus	Strabismus, nystagmus
• Red reflex	Present	Cataract
Child Testing • Visual acuity (Snellen Tumbling "E" chart [Fig. 9–7] for ages 3–7; not accurate < age 3).	Age 1: 20/200 Age 2: 20/70 Age 5: 20/30 Age 6: 20/20	Two-line difference between eyes 4-year-old with acuity of 20/40 or less
• Color differentiation check at age 5	Differentiates colors	Color blindness

G

PHYSICAL ASSESSMENT: EXTERNAL AND INTERNAL EYES

Geriatric Adaptations

Steps	Normal and/or Common Findings	Significant Deviations
Inspection • *Lids:* Note position.		Lid lag, ptosis, ectropion, entropion

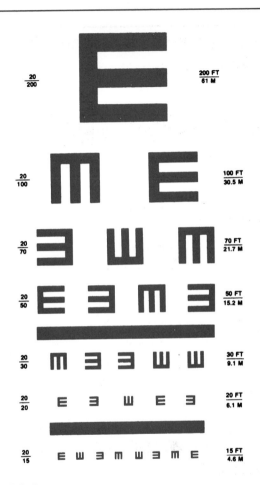

FIGURE 9–7

The Snellen Tumbling E chart. (*Source:* Adapted from Vision Screening Manual, Texas Department of Health, Austin, Texas, 1998, p 22, used with permission.)

G

PHYSICAL ASSESSMENT: EXTERNAL AND INTERNAL EYES (Continued)
Geriatric Adaptations

Steps	Normal and/or Common Findings	Significant Deviations
• Sclera: note color		Senile hyaline Plaque Arcus Senilis
• *Pupils:* Note size.	Diminished	
• *Cornea:* Note clarity.	Arcus senilis Diminished visual acuity Diminished adaptation to dark	Cloudy or opaque, abrasions, ulcerations
• *Lens:* Note clarity. *Test each eye separately.*	Clear	Cloudiness, opacity
Geriatric Testing		
• *Visual acuity Snellen chart:* Use lightened chart or a light behind the client. Test with and without corrective lenses.	20/20 to 20/30 with corrective lenses	Any line above the 20/30 line on the chart

R

PHYSICAL ASSESSMENT: EXTERNAL AND INTERNAL EYES
Racial and Ethnic Adaptations

Steps	Normal and/or Common Findings	Significant Deviations
Inspection • *Sclera:* Note color	Slight yellow cast Brown spots	Dots of pigmentation near corneal limbus

PHYSICAL ASSESSMENT: EXTERNAL AND INTERNAL EYES
Racial and Ethnic Adaptations

Steps	Normal and/or Common Findings	Significant Deviations
• *Eyeball:* Note position.	May protrude slightly beyond supraorbital ridge	
• Fundi (A-A)	Heavily pigmented uniformly dark	
• Conjunctivae		Pale
• Internal eye		Detached retina (severe sickle cell)

DIAGNOSTIC TESTS

May need to refer for:

- Mydriatic agent to dilate pupils for full fundoscopic exam
- Puff test for pressure in glaucoma

POSSIBLE NURSING DIAGNOSES

- Sensory-perceptual alterations, visual
- Social interaction, impaired
- Social isolation

Clinical Alert

- Explain possible discomfort of light and cotton wisp.
- Do not use light in eyes for excessively long times.
- If red reflex is absent, reposition scope.
- If client experiences sudden eye pain, large flashes of light, loss of vision, discharge, redness, or swelling, refer to an ophthalmologist as soon as possible.

SAMPLE DOCUMENTATION

Eyes: Symmetrical with no lag or turning of lids; no exophthalmos noted. Sclera clear, white; conjunctivae dark pink without inflammation. Irises light blue, intact. PERRLA. Extraocular muscles (EOMs) and normal visual fields intact (CN III, IV, VI). Alignment and convergence normal. Corneal reflex intact (CN V). Fundoscopic: Disks flat, yellow. No AV nicking, hemorrhage, or cupping noted; A3:V5. Acuity (CN II); OD 20/40, OS 20/20, OU 20/20. Corrected (Rosenbaum chart).

CLIENT AND FAMILY EDUCATION AND HOME HEALTH NOTES

Adult

- Recommend examination every 5 to 10 years until age 40, then every 2 to 5 years.
- Stress use of safety glasses with hobbies, home repair.

Pediatric

Infants

- Explain normal vision; that is, poor acuity and poor muscle control at birth, lack of tears until 3 months.

Children and Adolescents

- Use sunglasses when outdoors, especially when in the sun or in highly reflective area (e.g., sand, water, snow).
- Vision should be screened at ages 3, 4 to 6, 7 to 9, and 13.
- Color vision should be screened at 4 to 5 years of age.
- Use protective eyewear when performing hazardous activities.

Geriatric

- Explain drying of mucous membranes, possible need for artificial lubricants.
- Recommend examination every year and as necessary when changes occur.
- Emphasize that blindness caused by glaucoma or cataracts is preventable or treatable if detected early and that eye drops for glaucoma must be taken for a lifetime.
- Inform client of visual side effects of any medications being taken.
- Use bright, indirect lighting when performing fine tasks (reading, sewing).
- Use a magnifier for fine tasks if necessary.
- Inform client of the availablity of large-print books and reading materials.

- <u>Symptoms that require immediate attention:</u> Pain, discharge, redness or swelling, loss of vision, excessive tearing, floaters that occur in association with light flashes.

Racial and Ethnic

- Encourage testing for glaucoma every 1 to 2 years in African-Americans because of their high risk.
- Certain racial groups may respond differently to treatments (Jarvis, 2000).

ASSOCIATED COMMUNITY AGENCIES

- <u>American Society for the Blind:</u> Talking books, adaptive aids for the home
- <u>Foundation for Glaucoma Research:</u> Education and support
- <u>Lion's Club:</u> May provide glasses for children or adults
- <u>Local optometry schools:</u> Discounted eye exams
- <u>National Society to Prevent Blindness:</u> Information and local services such as eye exams
- <u>National Association for Parents of the Visually Impaired:</u> Provides support and promotes public understanding

CHAPTER 10

EARS

HISTORY

Adult

- Changes in hearing acuity, changes in speech sounds

- Aids to hearing used
- Vertigo, dizziness, earaches, drainage
- Exposure to loud sounds
- Medications affecting hearing, especially antibiotics
- Methods of hygiene
- History of renal disease, diabetes in self or family
- History of sinusitis, streptococcal infections
- History of Ménière's disease
- History of ear surgery, trauma

Pediatric
Infants

- Prematurity
- Maternal syphilis, rubella
- Exposure to antibiotics
- Chronic otitis media or upper respiratory infections
- Exposure to passive smoke
- Pulling or tugging at ears
- No increasing pattern of prespeech sounds/speech
- No reaction to loud noise
- Foul odor
- Allergies

Adolescents

- <u>Exposure to loud noises:</u> Chronic, acute, amount
- Frequency and sites of swimming
- Protrusion of external ear

ℂ **Geriatric**

- Hearing ringing or crackling noises
- Conversations of others sounding garbled or distorted
- Use of a hearing aid and its effectiveness
- Recurrent problems with cerumen impactions
- Frequently asking others to repeat themselves or keeping volume of radio or television turned up high
- Earache, dizziness, vertigo
- Hearing loss accompanied by suspiciousness, depression, social withdrawal, confusion
- Time of last audiometric examination
- Long-term exposure to loud noise

EQUIPMENT

- Otoscope
- Tuning fork
- Ticking watch
- Audiometer (if appropriate to setting)

CLIENT PREPARATION

- Client should be sitting.
- Tip head away from ear being examined.
- Parent may hold infant or toddler against parent's chest for otoscope exam.

PHYSICAL ASSESSMENT: EXTERNAL EAR

A

Adult

Steps	Normal and/or Common Findings	Significant Deviations
Inspection		
• Position of ear in relation to eye (Fig. 10–1)	Ear should be nearly upright, angling <10° toward occiput.	Unequal alignment, pinna below line level with corner of eye
• *Auricles:* Note size, shape, color, symmetry	Color of skin, uniform shape	Masses, lesions, deformities, cyanosis erythema, edema
Palpation		
• Earlobes	Smooth, uniform edge	Tophi, nodules
• Tragus, helix	Nontender	Tenderness, pain, ulcers
• Mastoid	Nontender	Edema, tenderness, masses
Testing Hearing Function: Test CN VIII		
• *Weber:* Place vibrating fork at midsagittal line (Fig. 10–2).	Client should hear or sense vibrations equally in both ears.	*Sound lateralized to one ear:* Perceptive loss from nerve damage, goes to unaffected ear. Conductive loss from otosclerosis, goes to affected ear.
• *Rinne:* Place vibrating fork on mastoid. After vibrations are no longer felt, hold fork beside ear to hear (see Fig. 10–2).	Air conduction = 2 × bone conduction; able to hear vibrations after feeling stops (air conduction greater than bone conduction).	If air conduction > 2 × bone conduction, there is perceptive loss. If air conduction < 2 × bone conduction, there is conductive loss.

Table continued on following page

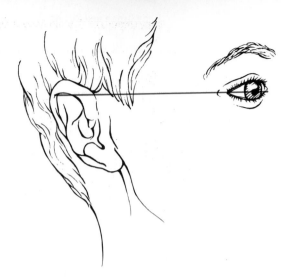

FIGURE 10–1
Position of eye and ear.

A PHYSICAL ASSESSMENT: EXTERNAL EAR

(Continued)
Adult

Steps	Normal and/or Common Findings	Significant Deviations
• Whisper test: Occlude one of client's ears and whisper 1–2 ft lateral to opposite ear.	Client should be able to hear half of all words whispered.	Unable to hear.
• Watch test. Start at about 18 in away from ear and compare with a person with normal hearing.	Able to hear at approximately the same distance as others with normal hearing are able to hear the same watch.	Unable to hear.

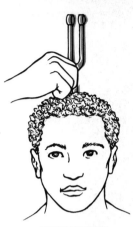

WEBER TEST

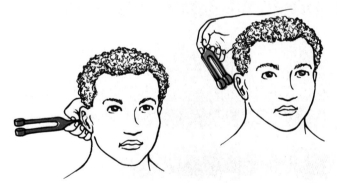

RINNE TEST

FIGURE 10–2
Weber test and Rinne test.

A

PHYSICAL ASSESSMENT: CANAL, MEMBRANE
Adult

Steps	Normal and/or Common Findings	Significant Deviations
Inspection • Anchor otoscope on client's head, tilted away from you; pull auricle up, out, and back to straighten auditory canal and *gently* insert speculum to depth of approximately ½ in (Fig. 10–3).		
• *Canal:* Note appearance of canal color; amount, type, and site of cerumen.	Moist brown cerumen, cilia.	Foreign bodies, discharge, lesions, foul odor, edema, flaking, erythema, moderate to severe pain on insertion
• *Tympanic membrane:* Note landmarks (umbo, cone of light, malleus handles), color (Fig. 10–4), integrity.	Silver-gray color, shiny, conical, intact. Old scars appear as white marks. Cone of light at 5 o'clock position in right ear and at 7 o'clock position in left ear.	Bulging (unable to note landmarks) or retracting (pronounced landmarks) Perforations, foul odor, discharge Dull, red, blue

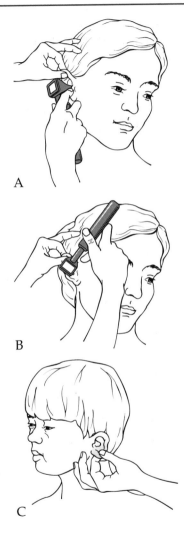

A

B

C

FIGURE 10–3
Use of otoscope. (*A, B*) Adult. (*C*) Child.

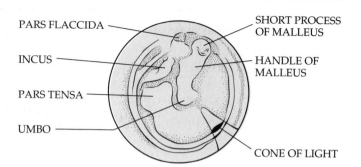

PARS FLACCIDA

INCUS

PARS TENSA

UMBO

SHORT PROCESS OF MALLEUS

HANDLE OF MALLEUS

CONE OF LIGHT

FIGURE 10–4

The tympanic membrane and landmarks of right ear.

PHYSICAL ASSESSMENT: EXTERNAL EAR, CANAL, MEMBRANE

Pediatric Adaptations
Infant

Steps	Normal and/or Common Findings	Significant Deviations
Inspection		
• *External:* Note shape and placement. Draw an imaginary line from the inner canthus of the eye to the outer canthus of the eye.	Uniform size and shape. Recoils briskly. Top of ear intersects this line.	Preauricular pits, dimples, skin tags Unusual shapes Low-set ears Slow or absent recoil Foul odor
• *Canal:* Stabilize head, restrain child firmly if needed, gently pull auricle down and back.	Vernix in canal (newborn).	Foreign body

158

PHYSICAL ASSESSMENT: EXTERNAL EAR, CANAL, MEMBRANE *(Continued)*

Pediatric Adaptations
Infant

Steps	Normal and/or Common Findings	Significant Deviations
• *Tympanic membrane:* Use pneumatic otoscope to differentiate from illness.	If membrane is red, may be caused by crying.	Fluid, edema, bulging, marked reddening Loss of bony landmarks Nonmobile tympanic membrane
Test • Infant	Flattened startle (Moro) or blink reflex.	Delayed or absent response
• 4–6 months old	Turns to sounds.	
• 8–10 months old	Responds to name.	
• 12 months old	Begins to imitate words.	
• *3–4 years old:* Use Weber or Rinne test		

PHYSICAL ASSESSMENT: EXTERNAL EAR, CANAL, MEMBRANE

Geriatric Adaptations

Steps	Normal and/or Common Findings	Significant Deviations
Inspection • *Auricles:* Note size.	Women may have large sagging lobes if they have worn heavy earrings for many years.	

Table continued on following page

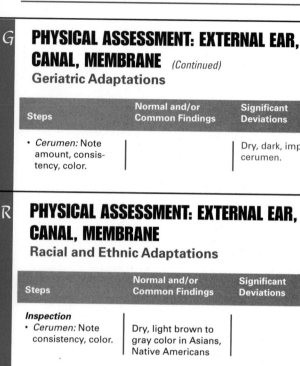

G PHYSICAL ASSESSMENT: EXTERNAL EAR, CANAL, MEMBRANE *(Continued)*
Geriatric Adaptations

Steps	Normal and/or Common Findings	Significant Deviations
• *Cerumen:* Note amount, consistency, color.		Dry, dark, impacted cerumen.

R PHYSICAL ASSESSMENT: EXTERNAL EAR, CANAL, MEMBRANE
Racial and Ethnic Adaptations

Steps	Normal and/or Common Findings	Significant Deviations
Inspection • *Cerumen:* Note consistency, color.	Dry, light brown to gray color in Asians, Native Americans	

DIAGNOSTIC TESTS

May need to refer to:

• Audiometric testing

POSSIBLE NURSING DIAGNOSES

• Communication, impaired verbal
• Social isolation
• Self-esteem disturbance
• Injury, risk for

Clinical Alert

- Refer to otolaryngologist for severe tenderness, pain, lesions, discharge, foreign bodies, and/or progressive hearing loss or ringing in the ears.

SAMPLE DOCUMENTATION

Verbal and nonverbal communication congruent and appropriate to setting. Auricles in alignment. Pinnae pink, elastic, symmetrical, without lesions, deformities, or tenderness. Auditory canals unobstructed, moderate amount of dark brown, moist cerumen present; tympanic membrane visualized intact, shiny and gray bilaterally; bony landmarks and light reflex present; no bulging, retractions, or redness. Vibratory sense intact; CN VIII intact with whisper test.

CLIENT AND FAMILY EDUCATION AND HOME HEALTH NOTES

Adult

- Do not attempt to clean or remove wax with a cotton swab or other device.
- Use washcloth or finger in outer ear.
- If canal needs cleaning, irrigate with bulb syringe, soaking with oil if necessary.
- Avoid excessively loud sounds or use ear plugs.

Pediatric

- Ear infections are common and potentially dangerous. Do not put to bed with bottles of milk or

161

other fluids. Be aware that colds and mild upper respiratory infections may develop into ear infections.

- Explain increased risk of otitis media for infants through preschoolers.
- Clean only outer ear using damp cloth.
- Child may insert objects into ears. Take child to health-care provider for removal of all objects.
- Eliminate exposure to smoke.
- Audiometric testing should be given to preschooler.
- Caution about loud music, especially when played through headphones.

Geriatric

- Have hearing tested annually by a physician or audiologist.
- Obtain a variety of hearing devices for the home, such as telephones with louder ringing mechanism and earpiece amplification, louder door chimes, wireless infrared TV listener.
- Do not be afraid to tell people to face you, speak at a slightly slower rate, use lower voice tones, be very clear, and do not shout.
- Teach how to care for hearing aids; explain that hearing aids should not be purchased unless recommended by a physician or audiologist. Purchase only from a reputable company (check with the Better Business Bureau).
  - Remove the hearing aid before going to bed, bathing, or showering.
  - Make sure the battery is inserted correctly. If there is no on-off switch, open the battery case at night to conserve the battery.

- Clean the ear mold daily with a damp cloth. Once a week, wipe the mold with a cloth dampened with mild, soapy water. If the hearing aid ear mold gets plugged with ear wax, <u>carefully</u> remove the wax with a toothpick or bent paperclip.

- Change the batteries every 10 days to 2 weeks. A whistle should be heard when the volume control is fully on.

- Remember, the aid makes sounds and voices louder, not clearer. Expectations should be realistic.

- Background noises may be annoying at first. Clients will most likely get used to the extraneous noise in a short time.

- If you are having any problems with the aid, have the aid tested by a reputable audiologist or hearing aid dealer.

ASSOCIATED COMMUNITY AGENCIES

- <u>American Speech-Language-Hearing Association:</u> Education, Helpline
- <u>American Tinnitus Association:</u> Self-help groups
- <u>Better Hearing Institute:</u> Hearing Helpline
- <u>National Association of the Deaf:</u> Information
- <u>National Information Center on Deafness:</u> Information on assistive devices
- <u>Self-Help for Hard of Hearing People, Inc.:</u> Information and support
- <u>American Society for Deaf Children</u>

CHAPTER 11
NOSE AND SINUSES
HISTORY

Adult
- Stuffiness, discharge: character, onset, duration, treatment
- Seasonality of symptoms
- Sore throat
- Infections
- Epistaxis: Cause, duration, treatment, associated symptoms
- Allergies; use of nose drops and/or sprays, antihistamines, decongestants
- Repeated sinus infections
- Changes in appetite, smell sense
- Cocaine use
- History of surgery and/or trauma
- Snoring, daytime sleepiness
- Chronic alcohol abuse

Pediatric
- Nasal quality of voice
- Horizontal nasal crease ("allergic salute")
- Rhinitis
- Playing with small objects near nose

Geriatric
- Constant drip from nose to throat
- Allergies, sneezing
- Pain

EQUIPMENT

- Penlight
- Nasal speculum

CLIENT PREPARATION

- Sitting

PHYSICAL ASSESSMENT: EXTERNAL
Adult

A

Steps	Normal and/or Common Findings	Significant Deviations
Inspection • *Nose:* Note shape, symmetry, color, discharge.	Varies Uniform, symmetrical, scant	Bullous, flaring, discharge (watery, purulent, mucoid, bloody), mucus, crusting
Palpation • *Nose:* Note masses, tenderness.	Straight, nontender	Masses, tenderness
• *Patency:* With client's mouth closed, occlude each naris to assess patency of opposite side.	Patent	Occluded
• *Frontal sinuses:* Press upward with thumbs under brow ridge.	Nontender	Tenderness, pain
• *Maxillary sinuses:* Press up with thumbs under zygomatic arch; press in over maxillary sinus.	Nontender	Tenderness, pain

Table continued on following page

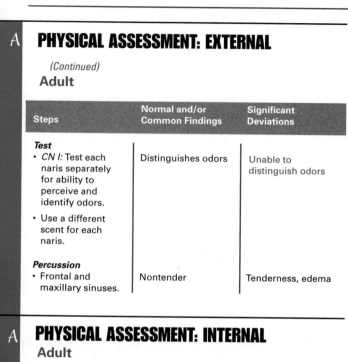

A | # PHYSICAL ASSESSMENT: EXTERNAL

(Continued)
Adult

Steps	Normal and/or Common Findings	Significant Deviations
Test • *CN I:* Test each naris separately for ability to perceive and identify odors.	Distinguishes odors	Unable to distinguish odors
• Use a different scent for each naris.		
Percussion • Frontal and maxillary sinuses.	Nontender	Tenderness, edema

A | # PHYSICAL ASSESSMENT: INTERNAL
Adult

Steps	Normal and/or Common Findings	Significant Deviations
Inspection • Tilt head back to insert speculum 1 cm. Avoid touching septum with speculum. • *Nares:* Note color, mucosa.	Pink and moist	Masses, lesions, redness, foreign bodies Polyps, fissures, ulcers, discharge, bleeding

PHYSICAL ASSESSMENT: INTERNAL

(Continued)
Adult

Steps	Normal and/or Common Findings	Significant Deviations
• *Inferior, middle, and superior turbinates:* Note color, consistency.	Pink, smooth (same-color as mucosa)	Redness, pallor, edema
• *Septum:* Note integrity, alignment.	Straight Uniform	Deviation due to trauma, bleeding

PHYSICAL ASSESSMENT: NOSE AND SINUSES

Pediatric Adaptations
Infant

Steps	Normal and/or Common Findings	Significant Deviations
Inspection • *Nose:* Note shape of bridge.	Straight	

Child

Steps	Normal and/or Common Findings	Significant Deviations
Inspection • *Nose:* Note horizontal crease. Note if mouth or nose breather.	No crease Breathes through nose	Flaring horizontal crease possible sign of allergies Consistently breathes through mouth; clearly audible breath sounds

Table continued on following page

P

PHYSICAL ASSESSMENT: NOSE AND SINUSES *(Continued)*
Pediatric Adaptations
Child

Steps	Normal and/or Common Findings	Significant Deviations
Palpation		
• Sphenoid, maxillary, ethmoid sinus (preschool child)	Nontender	Tender
• Frontal sinus (7–8 years of age)	Nontender	Tender

G

PHYSICAL ASSESSMENT: NOSE AND SINUSES
Geriatric Adaptations

Steps	Normal and/or Common Findings	Significant Deviations
Inspection		
• *Nose:* Note size.	Appears larger and more prominent with age	
Test		
• Sense of smell	Diminishes with age	Absent

PHYSICAL ASSESSMENT: NOSE AND SINUSES

Racial and Ethnic Adaptations

Steps	Normal and/or Common Findings	Significant Deviations
Inspection • *Nose:* Note shape, size.	Size and shape vary in different ethnic groups	

DIAGNOSTIC TESTS

May need to refer for

- Biopsy of suspicious lesions

POSSIBLE NURSING DIAGNOSES

- Breathing pattern, ineffective
- Injury, risk for
- Airway clearance, ineffective
- Aspiration, risk for
- Communication, impaired verbal

Clinical Alert

- **Prevent trauma to nasal mucosa with use of nasal speculum, nasal catheter, or nasogastric feeding tube.**

SAMPLE DOCUMENTATION

Nose aligned, symmetrical, without discharge or redness. Both nares patent, no tenderness or masses palpated. Mucosa and septum without redness, swelling, or lesions. Sinuses not tender. CN I intact; distinguishes aromas correctly.

CLIENT AND FAMILY EDUCATION AND HOME HEALTH NOTES

Adult

- Prevent trauma to sensitive mucous membranes of nose.

Pediatric

- Avoid insertion of foreign bodies into nose. If object has been inserted, take child to physician's office for removal if foreign body is not easily grasped.
- Demonstrate use of tissue and handwashing to prevent spread of upper respiratory infection (URI).

Geriatric

- If sense of smell is diminished, teach client to routinely check and turn off dials on gas stoves (to prevent asphyxiation) and to label with a specific date foods stored in the refrigerator (to prevent eating spoiled foods).
- Inspect pilot lights periodically to lessen risk of gas exposure.
- Have smoke detector installed in home and test every 6 months. Need detector that flashes light if person has major hearing deficit.

CHAPTER 12
MOUTH AND THROAT

HISTORY

Adult

- <u>Oral hygiene practices:</u> Method, products used, frequency
- <u>Dental apparatus:</u> Braces, dentures, bridges, or crowns
- Date of last dental exam
- Nutritional habits
- <u>Tobacco use:</u> Type, frequency, duration
- <u>Alcohol use:</u> Frequency, duration
- Pain
- Lesions
- Sore throat
- Hoarseness, change in voice
- Cough
- Difficulty chewing or swallowing
- History of herpes simplex, diabetes mellitus, periodontal disease, frequent streptococcal infections, tonsillectomy
- Medications that cause gum inflammation, for example, dilantin
- <u>Medications that diminish salivation:</u> Diuretics, antihistamines, anticholinergics, antihypertensives, antispasmodics, antidepressants

Pediatric

- Congenital defect
- Dental hygiene

- Number of teeth present
- Fluoridated water
- Use of bottle and/or pacifier
- Thumb sucking
- Sore throats

Geriatric

- Date of last dental exam
- Soreness or bleeding lips, gums, tongue, or throat
- Missing teeth or difficulty chewing
- If appropriate, state of repair and fit of dentures
- Dry mouth
- Alterations in taste
- Oral hygiene habits
- If dentures are used, note wearing habits, how old they are, how well they fit, and if they are in good repair.
- History of aspiration pneumonia. Symptoms of swallowing problems, such as frequent coughing and/or choking with eating and drinking, or drooling; delayed coughing noted after finished eating or drinking.

EQUIPMENT

- Light
- Gloves (clean)
- Gauze square
- Tongue depressor

CLIENT PREPARATION

- Sitting

PHYSICAL ASSESSMENT: MOUTH AND TONGUE

A

Adult

Steps	Normal and/or Common Findings	Significant Deviations
Inspection		
• *Lips:* Note color, symmetry, continuity at squamous-buccal junction (Fig. 12–1).	Pink, slight asymmetry, intact	Lesions, involuntary movement, cracks, fissures, drooping, cyanosis
• *Mucosa and gums:* Note color, integrity, adherence.	Pink, intact, moist	Redness, edema, lesions, masses, bleeding, cyanosis
• *Stenson's and Wharton's ducts:* Note color.	Smooth, pink	Redness, edema
• *Teeth:* Note number, color, hygiene.	Complete, white, clean	Multiple caries, missing teeth, fuzzy, dirty
• *Tongue:* Note size. Check lateral, dorsal, and ventral surfaces for color, coating, texture, vessels.	Fits comfortably in mouth with teeth together Pink to red with papillae present Midline fissures present Geographic tongue	Coated, white patches, pale, nodules, ulcers Papillae or fissures absent
• *Palate, oropharynx, uvula:* Note color, continuity, integrity.	Pink; hard palate firm with rugae, soft palate spongy, uvula in midline	Redness, edema, lesions, pigmented lesions Uvula deviated: Note direction. Softened hard palate
• *Tonsils:* Note color, size, discharge.	Pink to red 1+ to 2+	Exudate 3+ to 4+ Markedly reddened

Table continued on following page

173

A

PHYSICAL ASSESSMENT: MOUTH AND TONGUE *(Continued)*

Adult

Steps	Normal and/or Common Findings	Significant Deviations
Test		
• *CN XII:* Have client extend tongue and move side to side.	Tongue centrally aligned without fasciculations	No central alignment, fasciculations
• *CN IX, X:* Observe soft palate and uvula rising as client says "ah"; after alerting client, gently touch back of tongue with tongue depressor to elicit gag reflex.	Soft palate rising symmetrically, uvula in midline, quick gag reflex	Unequal or absent rise of soft palate; uvula deviated on rising Absent or diminished gag reflex
Palpate (Wearing gloves)		
• Check lips.		
• Assess gums.	Soft, smooth	Inflammation, edema, swelling, bleeding, receding from teeth
• *Tongue:* Ask client to protrude tongue; grasp tip with gauze square and gently pull to each side. Palpate sides of tongue.	Muscular Nontender, smooth Pink, moist, slightly rough Midline position Voluntary movement Symmetry of shape	Induration, lesions Tender, masses, redness Fasciculations Tumors
• Check teeth.	*Position and/or condition:* Stable, smooth	Loose, broken, irregular edges
Smell		
• Assess oral cavity.	No odor, tobacco, smoke, food odors	Foul, acetone, alcohol odor

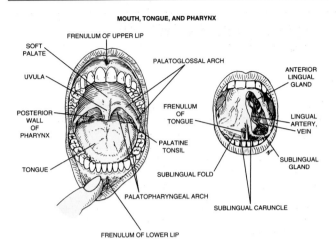

MOUTH, TONGUE, AND PHARYNX

FIGURE 12–1

Mouth, tongue, and pharynx. (*Source:* Taber's, 1997, ed 18, p 1237, with permission.)

PHYSICAL ASSESSMENT: MOUTH AND TONGUE

Pediatric Adaptations
Infant

Steps	Normal and/or Common Findings	Significant Deviations
Inspection • Assess oral cavity.	Pink Epstein's pearls, retention cysts	Thrush
• *Buccal mucosa:* Note amount and thickness of saliva, integrity of tissue.	Midline uvula, freely movable Small tonsils	Cyanosis Cleft palate, lip, or bifid uvula Excessive drooling in newborn

Table continued on following page

P

PHYSICAL ASSESSMENT: MOUTH AND TONGUE *(Continued)*

Pediatric Adaptations
Infant

Steps	Normal and/or Common Findings	Significant Deviations
• *Deciduous teeth:* Note number, development, eruption dates (Fig. 12–2).		
• *Tongue:* Note size.	Fits in mouth with teeth closed	Large, protruding Ankyloglossia
Palpate		
• Observe soft and hard palate.	Intact	Clefts

P

PHYSICAL ASSESSMENT: MOUTH AND TONGUE

Pediatric Adaptations
Child

Steps	Normal and/or Common Findings	Significant Deviations
Inspection		
• *Arch of palate:* Note color.	Koplik's spots	
• *Teeth:* Note number, color.	Malocclusion at age 8	No teeth by age 1
• *Tonsils:* Note size.	Hypertrophic in mid-childhood	Inflamed, red, edematous

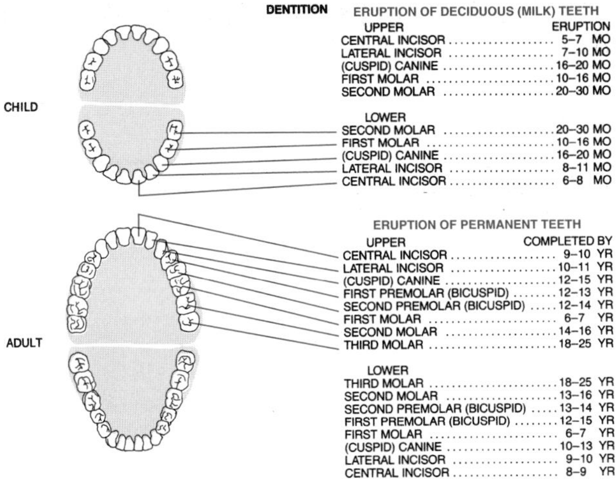

DENTITION	ERUPTION OF DECIDUOUS (MILK) TEETH

UPPER — ERUPTION

CENTRAL INCISOR .... 5–7 MO
LATERAL INCISOR .... 7–10 MO
(CUSPID) CANINE .... 16–20 MO
FIRST MOLAR .... 10–16 MO
SECOND MOLAR .... 20–30 MO

LOWER

SECOND MOLAR .... 20–30 MO
FIRST MOLAR .... 10–16 MO
(CUSPID) CANINE .... 16–20 MO
LATERAL INCISOR .... 8–11 MO
CENTRAL INCISOR .... 6–8 MO

ERUPTION OF PERMANENT TEETH

UPPER — COMPLETED BY

CENTRAL INCISOR .... 9–10 YR
LATERAL INCISOR .... 10–11 YR
(CUSPID) CANINE .... 12–15 YR
FIRST PREMOLAR (BICUSPID) .... 12–13 YR
SECOND PREMOLAR (BICUSPID) ..... 12–14 YR
FIRST MOLAR .... 6–7 YR
SECOND MOLAR .... 14–16 YR
THIRD MOLAR .... 18–25 YR

LOWER

THIRD MOLAR .... 18–25 YR
SECOND MOLAR .... 13–16 YR
SECOND PREMOLAR (BICUSPID) ..... 13–14 YR
FIRST PREMOLAR (BICUSPID) .... 12–15 YR
FIRST MOLAR .... 6–7 YR
(CUSPID) CANINE .... 10–13 YR
LATERAL INCISOR .... 9–10 YR
CENTRAL INCISOR .... 8–9 YR

FIGURE 12–2

Dentition (eruption of teeth). (*Source:* Taber's, 1997, ed 18, p 509, with permission.)

PHYSICAL ASSESSMENT: MOUTH AND TONGUE

P

Pediatric Adaptations
Adolescent

Steps	Normal and/or Common Findings	Significant Deviations
Inspection • *Teeth:* Note presence of 2nd and 3rd molars (see Fig. 12–2).		

G

PHYSICAL ASSESSMENT: MOUTH AND TONGUE

Geriatric Adaptations

Steps	Normal and/or Common Findings	Significant Deviations
Inspection		
• Lips	Smaller, decreased fat pad	Leukoplakia, lesions, **cracks in corners**
• Teeth	Darkened, worn down	Multiple obvious caries, **missing teeth**
• *Gums:* Ask client to remove dentures to see gums.	May be atrophied	Irritation, lesions, bleeding, inflammation, swelling, pyorrhea
• *Soft and hard palate:* Note color.	Pink Torus palatinus	Lesions
• Tongue	Fissures, varicosities on under surface	Extremely dry Thrush, lesions, deviations

R

PHYSICAL ASSESSMENT: MOUTH AND TONGUE

Racial and Ethnic Adaptations*

Steps	Normal and/or Common Findings	Significant Deviations
Inspection		
• *Lips:* Note surface integrity	African-American and Asian dimpling ≤4 mm at commissure. Size and shape vary in different ethnic groups.	

*Source: **Adapted from Jarvis, 2000.**

PHYSICAL ASSESSMENT: MOUTH AND TONGUE *(Continued)*
Racial and Ethnic Adaptations

Steps	Normal and/or Common Findings	Significant Deviations
• *Teeth:* Note size.	African American larger; Asian and Native American largest. Agenesis of third molars most frequent in Asians.	
• *Mucosa:* Note color integrity.	Hyperpigmentation.	Grayish white lesion
• *Palate and lingual mandible area:* Note surface.	Protuberances most common in Asians, Native Americans. Cleft palate and bifid uvula more common in Asians, Native Americans.	May interfere with dentures May indicate cleft palate.

DIAGNOSTIC TESTS

May need to refer for:

- Dental x-rays as needed
- Biopsy of suspicious lesions
- Throat cultures
- Swallowing studies

POSSIBLE NURSING DIAGNOSES

- Oral mucous membrane, altered
- Sensory-perceptual alteration, gustatory
- Nutrition: altered, less than body requirements
- Infection, risk for
- Aspiration, risk for

Clinical Alert

- Note severe signs of dehydration if lips, mucosa, and/or tongue are dry.

- Wear gloves to remove and clean dentures.

- Store dentures in a safe place when not in the client's mouth.

- Excess saliva may be aspirated.

- Bright red, +4 tonsils require prompt medical attention.

- Oral lesions, gingival erythema and edema, tooth decay or abscess—refer to a dentist.

- Observe for signs of swallowing difficulties, choking during eating or drinking, coughing 15 to 30 minutes after a meal, recurrent pneumonia, and drooling.

SAMPLE DOCUMENTATION

Adult

- Oral cavity pink, moist, smooth, clean. No missing or decaying teeth. Tonsils +1, without exudate or erythema. CN IX, X, XII intact. No masses or nodules palpated.

Pediatric

- Oral cavity pink and moist. Palate intact. Hypertrophic tonsils without redness or edema. Twenty deciduous teeth present without caries.

CLIENT AND FAMILY EDUCATION AND HOME HEALTH NOTES

Adult

- Client should brush with fluoride paste and floss between teeth at least at bedtime.

- Dilantin may cause gums to bleed. Clients on this medication should cleanse with very soft brush and floss gently. They should also consider having their teeth cleaned by a dentist more frequently than every 6 months.

- Remind clients with heart disease to inform dentist of their condition.

- Remind client to see dentist twice yearly for exam and professional cleaning. Clients who wear dentures should still see dentist every 6 months; this is necessary to check for oral cancers and problems in denture alignment. Note also that clients who have had a significant weight change should have a dentist check denture alignment.

- Remind client to limit sweets.

- Remind client to not smoke or chew tobacco.

Pediatric

- Caution parents to avoid prolonged exposure of mouth to milk or sweetened drinks (even before eruption of teeth). If bottle is taken to bed, it should contain only water. Bottles should <u>not</u> be propped in crib as there is a danger of aspiration in such circumstances.

- Discuss food safety with parents (e.g., aspiration, danger of straws).

- Explain to parents that they should use a spoon to feed baby cereal. Cereal should not be put in a bottle (aspiration hazard).

181

- Before teeth emerge, parents should wipe gums gently and often with damp, soft cloth.

- Brushing should begin with the first tooth. Parents may use infant toothbrush or a piece of gauze to clean teeth. Dental checkups should begin between ages 1 and 2; thereafter children should have checkups twice a year or yearly, as recommended by their dentist.

- Check fluoride level of drinking water for infants and children. Parents should check with dentist about taking fluoride tablets or using fluoride rinses. (Supplements are recommended if fluoride level in water <0.7 parts per million.)

- Reinforce dental hygiene guidelines for children between 7 to 10 years of age.

Geriatric

- If taste perception is decreased, encourage the use of spices such as cinnamon and garlic powder instead of extra salt and sugar.

- Explain that preventive oral care is a requirement across the life span.

- Encourage client to brush and floss teeth at least daily, preferably after each meal.

- Refer client to physician with any suspected problems with swallowing.

- Denture wearers:

  - Wear dentures during waking hours to prevent atrophy of gums.

  - See dentist if dentures do not fit properly and/or cause any irritation or pain to gums.

  - Brush dentures at least daily, preferably after each meal.

- Remove dentures at night and soak in water or a denture cleansing solution to prevent drying or warping.

- When caring for dentures, place a washcloth in the bottom of the sink in case dentures are accidentally dropped (will help prevent possible damage to the dentures).

- Rinse mouth thoroughly with warm water before replacing dentures in mouth after meals or in the morning.

Associated Community Agencies

- <u>Local dental or dental hygiene schools:</u> discounted exams

- <u>American Dental Association:</u> (free public education materials)

- <u>American Cleft Palate—Craniofacial Association</u>

CHAPTER 13

LUNGS AND THORAX

HISTORY

Adult

- Exposure to dust, chemicals and vapors, birds, asbestos, air pollutants

- Home environment, hobbies, travel

- <u>Allergies:</u> Type, response, treatments

- <u>Medications:</u> Prescription, OTC, illegal drugs

- <u>Tobacco use:</u> Type, duration, amount (packs, years), extent of passive smoking, years since quitting

- History of impaired mental status, exposure to infections
- <u>Cough:</u> Onset, type, duration, pattern, causes, severity, treatments
- Chest pain: Onset, duration, associated symptoms, treatments
- Shortness of breath: Onset, pattern, duration, causes, treatments
- Cyanosis or pallor
- History of emphysema, cancer, tuberculosis, heart disease, asthma, chest pain, allergies, sickle cell disease, immobility, obesity
- History of surgery, trauma
- Date of last chest x-ray and tuberculosis test
- Production of blood and/or other secretions with coughing
- Sedentary lifestyle, exercise intolerance
- Family history of tuberculosis, cystic fibrosis, asthma, emphysema, malignancy

Pediatric
Infants

- Immunizations (see App. H, Pediatric Immunization Schedule)
- Respiratory distress, cyanosis, apnea
- <u>SIDS:</u> Occurrence in sibling or other family member
- Exposure to passive smoke
- History of meconium ileus
- History of prematurity or mechanical ventilation
- Possible aspiration

- Difficulty feeding

Children

- Immunizations (see App. H, Pediatric Immunization Schedule)
- <u>Asthma history:</u> Associated factors related to episodes, treatment
- Frequent colds or congestion
- Swollen lymph nodes, sore throat, facial pain
- Night coughs

Geriatric

- History of annual influenza immunization
- History of pneumonia vaccine
- Recent change in exertional capacity, fatigue
- Significant weight changes
- Change in number of pillows used at night
- Painful breathing; night sweats; swelling of hands, ankles; tingling of arms or legs; leg cramps at rest or with movement
- Smoking history
- Difficulty swallowing with frequent respiratory infections

EQUIPMENT

- Stethoscope
- Tape measure
- Pen or washable marker
- Ruler
- Drapes

CLIENT PREPARATION

- Sitting

185

A

PHYSICAL ASSESSMENT: LUNGS AND THORAX
Adult

Steps	Normal and/or Common Findings	Significant Deviations
Inspection		
• *Shape:* Note anteroposterior (AP) to transverse ratio.	Approximately symmetrical, AP about 0.5 diameter of transverse	Barrel chest, pigeon chest, funnel chest
• Note color.		Cyanosis, pallor, especially of lips, nails, gums
• *Respiration:* Note rate, rhythm, depth, pattern.	12–20/min Expansion symmetrical	Distress; shallow, rapid; gasping; bradypnea, tachypnea; bulging or audible sounds; retractions
• *Fingers:* Note shape of nails.	Uniform	Clubbing (Fig. 13–1)
• Check lips.	No effort in breathing	Pursing
• Check nose.	No flaring	Flaring nares
Palpation		
• *Thorax:* Note tenderness, motion, pulsation, crepitus.	Approximate symmetry, firm shape, nontender, elastic motion No pulsations or crepitations	Pain, tenderness Crepitus (crinkly, crackles) Friction rub (coarse vibration, usually inspiratory)
• *Tactile fremitus:* Place palmar surface of fingers on auscultation sites simultaneously; ask client to repeat "99" while palpating; compare right and left sides.	Even, symmetrical Increased over major airways, decreased over lung bases	Decreased, absent, increased asymmetrical, coarsened Crepitus

Table continued on page 188

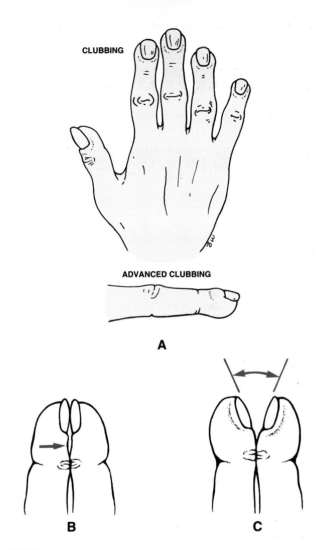

FIGURE 13–1

(*A*) Clubbing of fingers. (*Source:* Taber's, 1997, ed 18, p 401, with permission.) (*B*) Normal nails with arch illustrated by arrow. (*C*) Clubbed nails with arrow illustrating loss of arch and exaggerated angle. (*Source:* Adapted from Seidel et al, Mosby's Guide to Physical Examination, ed 4. Mosby, St. Louis, 1999, p 186, with permission.)

A

PHYSICAL ASSESSMENT: LUNGS AND THORAX *(Continued)*
Adult

Steps	Normal and/or Common Findings	Significant Deviations
• Expansion (thumbs at 10th rib) (Fig. 13–2).	Symmetrical expansion of 2–3 in	Asymmetrical expansion <2 in
Percussion • *Thorax:* Compare left and right; note tone, intensity, pitch.	(See Table 4–2.) *Flat:* Large muscles, viscera, bones *Dull:* Heart, liver *Tympany:* Stomach *Resonance:* All of lung field	Hyperresonance Dullness Hyperresonance, tympany, dullness, flatness over lung tissue
• Measure diaphragmatic excursion. Percuss downward in midscapular line as client holds deep inspiration, from resonance to dullness. Mark lower border where dullness begins. Ask client to exhale completely, then percuss upward from mark to beginning of resonance. Mark and measure. Repeat on other side.	3–5 cm; may be higher on right	No change or decrease Increased excursion
Auscultation • (Ask client to breathe fairly deeply through mouth.)	Vesicular, over lung field, inspiration > expiration; bronchovesicular over	Bronchovesicular or bronchial breath sounds over peripheral lung fields

Table continued on page 190

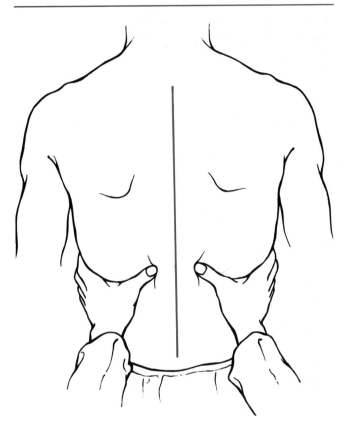

FIGURE 13–2
Measurement of thoracic expansion.

A PHYSICAL ASSESSMENT: LUNGS AND THORAX *(Continued)*

Adult

Steps	Normal and/or Common Findings	Significant Deviations
Auscultate with diaphragm, through complete inspiration and expiration, at each site, (Figs. 13–3 through 13–5) as client crosses arms over chest and leans forward. Compare bilaterally. Note pitch, intensity, duration of inspiration and expiration (Fig. 13–6), and any adventitious sounds (Fig. 13–7).	main stem bronchi, inspiration = expiration; bronchial over trachea, inspiration < expiration	Diminished, absent, markedly increased breath sounds, adventitious sounds; crackles (rales), wheezes, gurgles (ronchi), friction
• *Cough:* Note moisture, pitch, quality, frequency.	No cough	Cough with yellow, pink, brown, or gray sputum

P PHYSICAL ASSESSMENT: LUNGS AND THORAX

Pediatric Adaptations
  Infant

Steps	Normal and/or Common Findings	Significant Deviations
Inspection • Note respiration rate.	30–60 (newborn), 22–40 (by 1 year old)	

Table continued on page 192

190

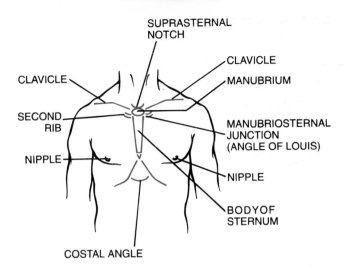

FIGURE 13-3
Topographic landmarks of chest.

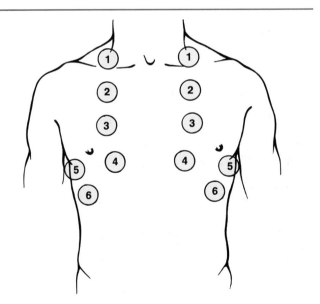

FIGURE 13-4
Anterior thoracic auscultation and palpation sites.

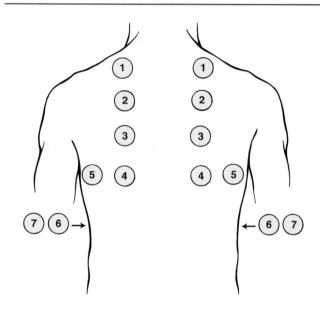

FIGURE 13–5

Posterior thoracic auscultation, percussion, and palpitation sites.

PHYSICAL ASSESSMENT: LUNGS AND THORAX *(Continued)*

Pediatric Adaptations
Infant

Steps	Normal and/or Common Findings	Significant Deviations
• *Shape:* Note chest and head circumference.	Approximately equal in neonate Abdominal breathing	Unequal chest expansion Paradoxical breathing
• Note AP and transverse diameter.	Approximately equal	

Table continued on page 195

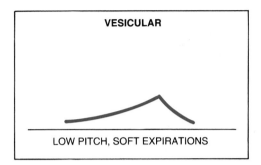

VESICULAR

LOW PITCH, SOFT EXPIRATIONS

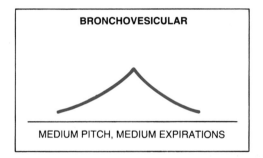

BRONCHOVESICULAR

MEDIUM PITCH, MEDIUM EXPIRATIONS

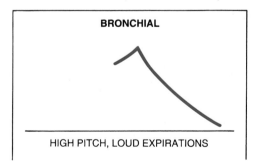

BRONCHIAL

HIGH PITCH, LOUD EXPIRATIONS

FIGURE 13–6

Normal breath sounds. (*Source:* Adapted from Thompson, JM, et al: Mosby's Clinical Nursing, ed 3. Mosby, St. Louis, 1993, p 136, with permission.)

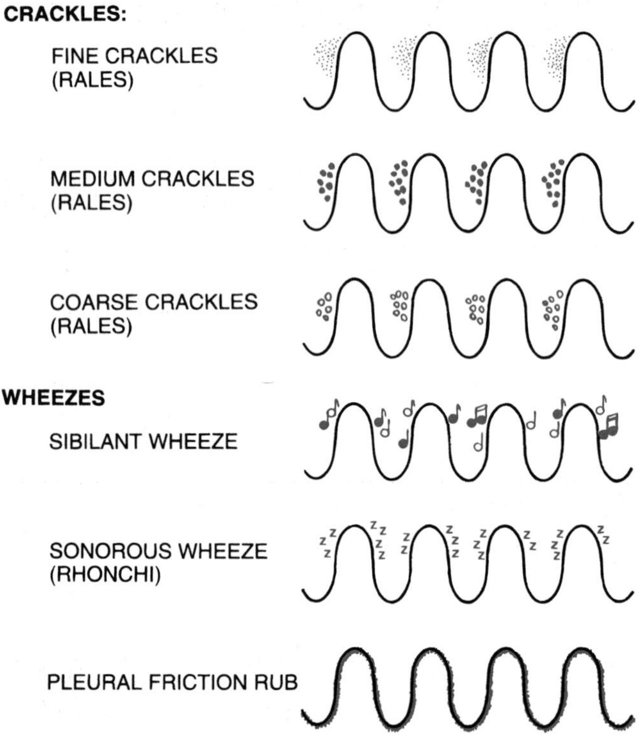

CRACKLES:

FINE CRACKLES
(RALES)

MEDIUM CRACKLES
(RALES)

COARSE CRACKLES
(RALES)

WHEEZES

SIBILANT WHEEZE

SONOROUS WHEEZE
(RHONCHI)

PLEURAL FRICTION RUB

FIGURE 13–7

Abnormal breath sounds. (*Source:* Adapted from Thompson, JM, et al: Mosby's Clinical Nursing, ed 3. Mosby, St. Louis, 1993, p 137, with permission.)

PHYSICAL ASSESSMENT: LUNGS AND THORAX *(Continued)*

P

Pediatric Adaptations
Infant

Steps	Normal and/or Common Findings	Significant Deviations
• Note respiratory pattern.	Diaphragmatic breather	Retractions, nasal flaring, periodic breathing, apnea, grunting, stridor
Auscultation		
• Check lung fields.	Loud, equal	Muffled, unequal, hyperresonant, diminished

PHYSICAL ASSESSMENT: LUNGS AND THORAX

P

Pediatric Adaptations
Child

Steps	Normal and/or Common Findings	Significant Deviations
Inspection		
• Shape	Should approximate adult shape, uniform	Barrel chest Pectus carinatum Pectus excavatum
• Rate	Approximately: 26 by age 4 20 by age 10 16 by age 16	

G PHYSICAL ASSESSMENT: LUNGS AND THORAX

Geriatric Adaptations

Steps	Normal and/or Common Findings	Significant Deviations
Inspection • *Thoracic spine:* Note curvature, angles.	Essentially straight	Marked dorsal curvature, kyphosis, increased AP diameter of chest
• Assess chest expansion.		Diminished

R PHYSICAL ASSESSMENT: LUNGS AND THORAX

Racial and Ethnic Adaptations

Steps	Normal and/or Common Findings	Significant Deviations
Inspection • Note position while breathing.		Arching back to ease dyspnea in sickle cell crisis
Auscultation • Look for signs of cor pulmonale.		Productive cough, exertional dyspnea, wheezing, fatigue, dependent edema, weak rapid pulse

DIAGNOSTIC TESTS

May need to refer for:

- Chest x-ray
- TB tine test
- Culture and sensitivity of sputum
- Modified barium swallow

POSSIBLE NURSING DIAGNOSES

- Airway clearance, ineffective
- Breathing pattern, ineffective
- Suffocation, risk for
- Tissue perfusion, altered: cardiopulmonary
- Gas exchange, impaired
- Infection, risk for

Clinical Alert

- **Persistent or paroxysmal cough**
- **Cyanosis**
- **Air hunger, dyspnea**
- **Hemoptysis**
- **Stridor**

SAMPLE DOCUMENTATION

Color pink without cyanosis or pallor. Respiration 16, regular, even depth. Chest equal symmetrically; AP diameter is half transverse. Tactile fremitus and thoracic expansion symmetrical and equal. All lung fields resonant equally. Vesicular sounds throughout; no adventitious sounds auscultated.

CLIENT AND FAMILY EDUCATION AND HOME HEALTH NOTES

Adult

- Educate about smoking hazards, indoor pollution, exposure to respiratory irritants.
- Offer literature on quitting smoking, effective breathing patterns and coughing awareness, controlled breathing techniques.
- Be sure college students have had second measles-mumps-rubella vaccination.

Pediatric

- Educate parents regarding importance of immunizations.
- Instruct parents in risks associated with passive smoking.
- Instruct parents in use of vaporizer or humidifier.
- Educate parents on importance of handwashing to prevent spread of viral infections.
- Caution parents about the risks of infants and small children aspirating foreign objects, foods, and toy parts.
- Explain hazards of choking associated with adding cereal to bottles and/or propping bottles in the crib.
- Encourage parents to take CPR class.
- Discuss swimming safety issues.
- Instruct parents to position infant on back or side unless prohibited by other medical problems.

Geriatric

- Instruct clients to avoid environments where there are persons with respiratory infections.
- Instruct clients to avoid noxious fumes.
- Note that infection may occur without a major increase in temperature or presence of a severe cough.
- Note that most older persons should have pneumonia and influenza vaccinations. Only one pneumonia vaccination is necessary in a lifetime (recommended at age 65) unless client received the 14-valent vaccine before 1983 or is at high risk for respiratory problems, in which case another vaccination may be needed 5 or 6 years after the first. Influenza vaccinations are necessary yearly. If client is immunosuppressed or has a chronic disease, he or she may need influenza or pneumococcal vaccinations before 65. Health-care workers should receive influenza vaccinations before age 65.
- Raising the head and shoulders on several pillows can help persons breathe better when they feel dyspneic.
- Refer clients to physician in case of persistent cough.

Clinical Alert

Refer any person with a persistent or productive cough, new or increased dyspnea, orthopnea, or painful breathing.

Associated Community Agencies

- <u>American Lung Association:</u> Health promotion information, better breathing club, asthma camp

- <u>Office on Smoking and Health:</u> Information and publications

- <u>American Cancer Society:</u> Provides hospital beds and other adaptive aids for cancer clients, helps finance prescriptions for cancer treatment, health promotion information

- <u>Cystic Fibrosis Foundation</u>

- <u>National Foundation for Asthma</u>

CHAPTER 14

BREASTS AND AXILLAE

HISTORY

Adult

- Age at menarche, menopause

- Age during pregnancies, breast-feeding

- Use of hormonal medications, oral contraceptives, hormone replacement therapy

- <u>Breast self-examination:</u> How often, method used

- <u>Mammogram:</u> Date, findings

- Breast surgery, trauma, or disease

- <u>Change in breast:</u> Lumps, discharge, shape, skin, lesions, erythema swelling, tenderness, change in position of nipple, nipple discharge or inversion, relationship of breast changes to menses

- <u>Breast cancer, self, family:</u> Age at diagnosis, treatment, response

- <u>Lumps:</u> Size, location, how long, tenderness, relationship to menses

- Rash or eczema on nipples
- Fat and caffeine intake
- Risk factors for breast cancer:
  - Age >40, female
  - Early menarche, late menopause, chronically irregular menses untreated
  - Nulliparity
  - Over age 30 with first pregnancy
  - Previous breast cancer
  - Ovarian, uterine, or bowel cancer
  - Medications to suppress lactation
  - Breast cancer in mother, sister, aunt, grandmother, daughter
  - High intake of dietary fat
  - Postmenopausal weight gain

Pediatric

- Age at thelarche
- Adolescent boys: Unilateral or bilateral enlargement of breasts

Geriatric

- Prescription medications that may cause gynecomastia in older men
- Breast self-examinations
- Recent changes in breast characteristics
- Injury to breast tissue

EQUIPMENT

- Small pillow
- Measuring tape
- Small sheet or towel

CLIENT PREPARATION

Adult

- Client should be sitting and may need to stand and bend forward.
- Maintain privacy.

Pediatric

- Explain normal process of physical and sexual development.
- Tell child findings are normal.

PHYSICAL ASSESSMENT: BREASTS AND AXILLAE

Adult

Steps	Normal and/or Common Findings	Significant Deviations
Inspection • Repeat in three positions for women, sitting position only for men; sitting, arms at side; sitting, arms raised over head; sitting, hand on hips, pushing in. If breasts are very large, have client stand, bend forward at waist; inspect for shape and contour.		
• Shape.	Conical to pendulous	Marked difference in contour
• Size, symmetry.	Generally equal	Marked differences

PHYSICAL ASSESSMENT: BREASTS AND AXILLAE *(Continued)*

A

Adult

Steps	Normal and/or Common Findings	Significant Deviations
• Contour.	Symmetrical	Retraction, dimpling, flattening
• Color.	Light, striae Darkened areola	Redness
• Venous pattern.	Symmetrical, faint	Superficial dilation, asymmetrically increased pattern
• Texture.	Smooth, soft	Lesions, peau d'orange appearance
• Nipple, areolar tissue.	Lifetime inversion, Montgomery tubercles, supernumerary nipples	Retraction, deviation, rashes, discharge, recent inversion
Palpation *• Repeat in two positions for women:* Sitting arms at sides; supine, small pillow under shoulder of side being palpated. Omit supine position for men. Follow either clock or wedge pattern, using pads of three fingers (Figs. 14–1 through 14–3). Palpate breast and axillae.		
• Consistency.	Varies	Thickening, masses
• Tenderness.	Tender if premenstrual	Pain

Table continued on following page

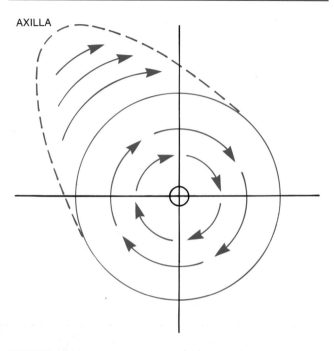

FIGURE 14–1

A palpation method for the breast and tail of Spence.

A

PHYSICAL ASSESSMENT: BREASTS AND AXILLAE *(Continued)*
Adult

Steps	Normal and/or Common Findings	Significant Deviations
• *Nodules:* Note location, size, shape, consistency, delimitation, mobility, tenderness.	None	Masses, areas of induration

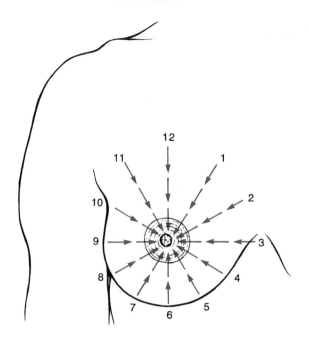

FIGURE 14–2
Clock pattern of breast examination.

PHYSICAL ASSESSMENT: BREASTS AND AXILLAE *(Continued)*
Adult

Steps	Normal and/or Common Findings	Significant Deviations
• *Nipples:* Gently compress.	No discharge	Discharge
• *Lymph nodes:* Lateral, subscapular, pectoral, central. Note presence, location, size, delimitation, shape, consistency, mobility, tenderness.	None	Palpable

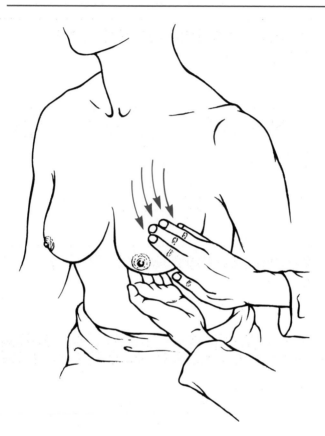

FIGURE 14–3

Bimanual palpation of the breast: technique used for large, pendulous breasts.

PHYSICAL ASSESSMENT: BREASTS AND AXILLAE

Pediatric Adaptations
Infant

Steps	Normal and/or Common Findings	Significant Deviations
Inspection • *Breasts:* Note size, discharge.	Nonpalpable, no discharge. Engorgement <1.5 cm, scant milky discharge in newborns; supernumerary nipples.	

PHYSICAL ASSESSMENT: BREASTS AND AXILLAE

Pediatric Adaptations
Child

Steps	Normal and/or Common Findings	Significant Deviations
Inspection • *Breast:* Note size, symmetry.	Breast development after age 8. May be asymmetrical (Table 14–1).	
Palpation • *Breast:* Note tenderness, masses.	Boys may have small, tender breast buds. Tender.	Masses Gynecomastia

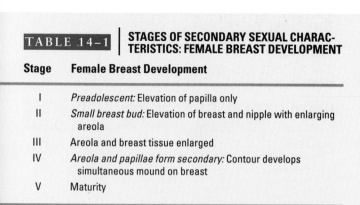

TABLE 14-1	STAGES OF SECONDARY SEXUAL CHARAC-TERISTICS: FEMALE BREAST DEVELOPMENT

Stage	Female Breast Development
I	*Preadolescent:* Elevation of papilla only
II	*Small breast bud:* Elevation of breast and nipple with enlarging areola
III	Areola and breast tissue enlarged
IV	*Areola and papillae form secondary:* Contour develops simultaneous mound on breast
V	Maturity

Source: Data from Tanner, JM: Growth at Adolescence, ed 2. Blackwell Scientific Publications, Oxford, England, 1962.

G

PHYSICAL ASSESSMENT: BREASTS AND AXILLAE
Geriatric Adaptations

Steps	Normal and/or Common Findings	Significant Deviations
Inspection		
• *Breasts:* Note size, shape, lesions, color, nodules.	Loose, atrophied, pendulous	Redness, irritation under breast, dimpling, masses
• *Nipples:* Note size, direction.	Flat, small	Dimpling, recent or new inversion, masses, discharge

DIAGNOSTIC TESTS

May need to refer for:

- Mammogram
- Biopsy

POSSIBLE NURSING DIAGNOSES

- Tissue integrity, impaired
- Body image disturbance
- Self-esteem disturbance
- Anxiety

Clinical Alert

Refer any suspicious lump, skin changes, dimpling, new nipple inversion or nipple discharge, or unusual breast discomfort.

SAMPLE DOCUMENTATION

Adult

- Breasts symmetrical, small, without lesions; texture smooth. No discharge or tenderness of nipple or areola. Nipples everted bilaterally. No masses or tenderness palpable in any region of breast or tail of Spence. No axillary or epitrochlear nodes palpable.

Infant

- Nipples symmetrical. No discharge. No masses.

Child
- Tanner stage II. No discharge. No masses or tenderness.

CLIENT EDUCATION AND HOME HEALTH NOTES

Adult
- Assess client's understanding of breast cancer, history, prevention, and early detection.
- Instruct both male and female clients in BSE (Fig. 14–4).
- Explain importance of regular breast exam performed by a health professional.
- Explain risks of large intake of caffeine and fat in breast cancer.
- Explain importance of mammogram and suggested schedule: once between ages 35 and 40, every year or every other year between ages 40 and 50, and every year after age 50 (more frequently if at risk).
- Explain incidence of recovery related to cancer.
- Encourage questions.

Pediatric
Infants
- Explain influence of maternal hormones to parents if infant has palpable breast tissue.

Children
- Explain patterns of breast development.
- Reassure adolescent boys with breast enlargement that condition is temporary.
- Teach BSE.

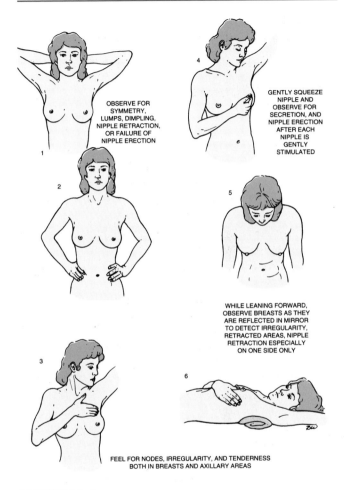

FIGURE 14–4

Breast self-examination. (*Source:* Taber's, 1997, ed 18, p 262, with permission.)

211

Geriatric
- Explain the importance of monthly BSE at set date every month after menopause (e.g., the first day of the month).
- Encourage client to continue mammogram screening.

ASSOCIATED COMMUNITY AGENCIES
- American Cancer Society

CHAPTER 15

CARDIOVASCULAR SYSTEM

HISTORY

Adult
- <u>Tobacco use:</u> Age started, type, amount (pack-years), duration, years since quitting.
- <u>Exercise habits:</u> Amount, type, duration, response.
- <u>Nutrition:</u> Usual diet; fat, salt, cholesterol, calorie intake.
- <u>Weight:</u> Recent change, percent obese. Optimal weight for adult female is 100 lb plus 5 lb for every inch above 5 ft tall (Edelman and Mandle, 1998). Adult males should weigh 110 lb plus 5 lb for every inch above 5 ft tall. Obesity is defined as 20 lb over ideal weight (see App. R for a weight table).
- <u>Alcohol use:</u> Amount, frequency.
- Stress management skills, ability, and methods used to relax; response to pressure, anger.
- Self or family history of heart disease, diabetes, rheumatic fever, hyperlipidemia, hypertension, early deaths, congenital heart defects.

- Presence or history of chest pain: **Onset, duration, severity, characteristics, associated symptoms, treatment, response.**
- Shortness of breath.
- Recent increase in fatigue, inability to complete usual activities.
- Dyspnea, orthopnea.
- Cough.
- Leg cramps: Onset (daily activities, awake at night), duration, characteristics.
- Extremities: Coldness, tingling, numbness, cyanosis, lesions, varicosities, slowed healing, edema.
- Medication use: Prescription and OTC.
- Syncope.

Pediatric
Infants

- Unusual fatigue, effort, or diaphoresis especially when feeding
- Circumoral cyanosis
- Coordination problems
- Generalized cyanosis (especially when crying)
- Breathing changes
- Mother's health during pregnancy (rubella: first trimester, unexplained fever, drug use)

Children

- Unusual fatigue: Amount, degree, activity level, need for rest, naps longer than expected
- Assumption of squatting or knee-chest position when playing
- Difficulty feeding

- Complaints of leg pain, joint pain, headache
- Nosebleeds
- Frequent streptococcal infections or sore throat with fever
- Headaches

Geriatric

- Chest pain, chest pressure, chest tightness
- Unusual fatigue, increased need for rest
- <u>Orthopnea:</u> Excessive number of pillows
- Shortness of breath, dyspnea, coughing, wheezing
- Dizziness, syncope, palpitations, confusion
- Use of cardiac or hypertensive medications
- Pounding heart with stress
- <u>Dietary history:</u> Intake of potassium, cholesterol, caffeine
- Nocturia
- <u>Foot and leg edema:</u> Tightness of shoes at end of day
- Change in exercise level
- Use of restrictive clothing
- Shortness of breath at night
- Peripheral vascular complaints such as coldness, decreased pain sensation, exaggerated response to cold, lower extremity fatigue/discomfort that worsens with walking or resting leg pain

Racial and Ethnic

- Sickle cell disease; associated subjective signs of pain, lethargy, dyspnea, low-grade fever

EQUIPMENT

- Stethoscope with diaphragm and bell
- Centimeter ruler
- Light
- Scale

The assessment of blood pressure is a part of assessing the cardiac system, but it is found in the vital signs section (see pages 87, 89, and 91).

CLIENT PREPARATION

Adult
- Remove clothing; drape well for warmth and privacy.
- Positions: Primarily sitting; also supine, left lateral recumbent, standing.

Pediatric
- A quiet child and a quiet environment are important.
- Use a pacifier to quiet an infant.
- Allow parent to hold child.

A
PHYSICAL ASSESSMENT: HEART
Adult

Steps	Normal and/or Common Findings	Significant Deviations
Inspection • Precordium movement with tangential lighting. • Jugular vein. • General muscle mass.	Slight apical impulse at midclavicular line (MCL), 5th intercostal space (ICS)	Marked pulsations; often not visible; impulse visible in more than one ICS or lateral to MCL; pulsations in other locations; heaves, lifts
Palpation • Lightly palpate precordium. Note location, strength of apical impulse.	Mild sensation palpable at 5th LICS, MCL	Thrills, pulsations Palpable in radius >1–2 cm or significantly to left or right of MCL or upward
• Palpate carotid and apical impulse simultaneously.	Synchronous pulses	
Auscultation • Auscultate in each of five areas (Fig. 15–1). Sitting, with diaphragm; supine, with both diaphragm and bell.	Synchronous pulses	
• Note rate, rhythm, location, and nature of S_1, S_2.	Normal sinus rhythm. S_1 loudest at apex. S_2 at base. Splitting of S_1 usually heard at left lower sternal border (tricuspid area); splitting of S_2 usually heard during inspiration at 2nd or 3rd left intercostal space (LICS).	S_3, S_4 audible at apex on inspiration Extra heart sounds such as clicks, snaps, friction rubs

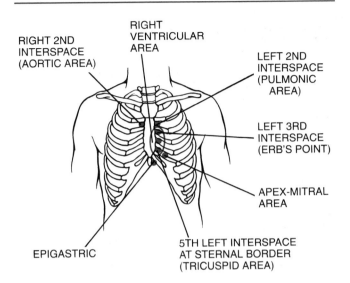

FIGURE 15–1

Cardiac auscultation and palpation sites.

PHYSICAL ASSESSMENT: HEART *(Continued)*
Adult

Steps	Normal and/or Common Findings	Significant Deviations
• Auscultate along left sternal border at 2nd and 3rd ICS (pulmonic area) with diaphragm as client leans forward. With client in left lateral recumbent position, auscultate at 5th LICS (mitral area) with bell.	No murmurs.	Murmurs. Note if increased on inspiration or expiration, with Valsalva maneuver, with elevation of legs, or if associated with diastole or systole. (Table 15–1).

TABLE 15–1	CLASSIFICATION OF MURMURS
Classification	**Murmur**
Grade I	Faint
Grade II	Heard fairly well in all positions
Grade III	Loud, no thrills
Grade IV	Loud, with a thrill
Grade V	Very loud, easily palpable thrill
Grade VI	May be heard without a stethoscope; thrill present

A PHYSICAL ASSESSMENT: PERIPHERAL CIRCULATION

Adult

Steps	Normal and/or Common Findings	Significant Deviations
Inspection • *Skin of extremities:* Note color, continuity, edema, vascularity.	Pink, no edema, no lesions	Cyanosis, lesions, ulcers, **varicosities,** edema, rubor
Palpation • Palpate carotid pulses (one at a time).	Symmetrical, rate 60–100 beats per minute, regular rhythm	Unequal, marked bradycardia, tachycardia, arrhythmias such as bigeminal pulse, alternating pulse, bounding or absent pulse

PHYSICAL ASSESSMENT: PERIPHERAL CIRCULATION *(Continued)*
Adult

A

Steps	Normal and/or Common Findings	Significant Deviations
• Palpate peripheral pulses bilaterally (Fig. 15–2): • Brachial • Radial • Femoral • Popliteal • Dorsalis pedis • Posterior tibial Note rate, rhythm, strength, symmetry; compare side to side.		
• Palpate extremities. Note temperature, tenderness, turgor, texture, hair growth, nails, varicosities, lesions, capillary refill time.	Warm; nontender; firm without edema; equal, fine hair growth; no lesions or varicosities, capillary refill <2 seconds	Cool, tender, pitting edema (0 to +4), absence of hair, varicose veins
• Measure jugular venous pressure. Place client in supine position with 45-degree elevation of head and shoulders. Observe jugular pulsation. With centimeter ruler, measure between highest point of jugular pulsation and angle of Louis	≤2 cm; usually absent on persons <age 50	>2 cm

Table continued on following page

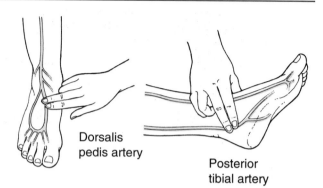

Dorsalis
pedis artery

Posterior
tibial artery

A. Palpation of dorsalis
pedis artery

B. Palpation of posterior
tibial pulse

FIGURE 15–2
Palpation of peripheral pulses.

A. **PHYSICAL ASSESSMENT: PERIPHERAL CIRCULATION** *(Continued)*
Adult

Steps	Normal and/or Common Findings	Significant Deviations
(Fig. 15–3). Mark the jugular pressure point with a straightedge for ease of measuring. Repeat on other side.		
Auscultation • *Auscultate with bell:* Temporal, carotid.	No audible sounds	Bruits

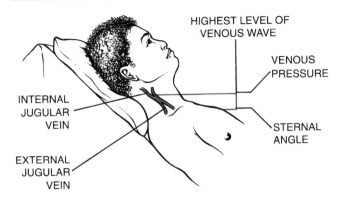

FIGURE 15–3
Inspection of jugular vein.

PHYSICAL ASSESSMENT: HEART AND PERIPHERAL CIRCULATION

Pediatric Adaptations
Infant

Steps	Normal and/or Common Findings	Significant Deviations
Inspection • *Apical impulse:* Note location.	4th LICS medial to MCL (<5 years old)	On right side may indicate situs inversus, heave
Palpation • Apical impulse		Thrills
• *Femoral and brachial pulses:* Note symmetry.	Equal bilaterally	Bounding Absent or weak in lower extremities
• Note capillary refill.	1–2 seconds	>2 seconds

Table continued on following page

221

PHYSICAL ASSESSMENT: HEART AND PERIPHERAL CIRCULATION *(Continued)*

Pediatric Adaptations
Infant

Steps	Normal and/or Common Findings	Significant Deviations
Auscultation • *Heart sounds:* Note rate, rhythm, location, nature of S_1, S_2, S_3.	Sinus arrhythmia	Machinelike continuous murmur, bradycardia, tachycardia

PHYSICAL ASSESSMENT: HEART AND PERIPHERAL CIRCULATION

Pediatric Adaptations
Child

Steps	Normal and/or Common Findings	Significant Deviations
Inspection • Apical impulse medial to left MCL at 4th ICS in child <5 years old	*Heart rate:* 1 year old: 80–140 3 years old: 80–120 5 years old: 75–110 10 years old: 70–100 Sinus arrhythmia	
Auscultation • *Heart sounds:* Sitting and supine	Splitting of S_2 at apex; innocent murmurs, grade 3 or less, present in systole; varying with respirations, found along left sternal border with child supine	No splitting of S_2 during inspiration.

PHYSICAL ASSESSMENT: HEART AND PERIPHERAL CIRCULATION *(Continued)*

Pediatric Adaptations
Child

Steps	Normal and/or Common Findings	Significant Deviations
• *Blood pressure:* All four extremities	Equal	Discrepancy between BP in upper and lower extremities may be indicative of coarctation of the aorta.

P

PHYSICAL ASSESSMENT: HEART AND PERIPHERAL CIRCULATION

Geriatric Adaptations

Steps	Normal and/or Common Findings	Significant Deviations
Inspection • Feet, toes, extremities	Varicose veins may appear when legs are in dependent position. Veins should collapse when elevated. Nails thicken; hair thins.	Rubor, lesions, marked edema, persistent cyanosis, venous stasis, brown skin, color changes, marked pallor, delayed color return, *resting* leg pain, nonhealing ulcers, pain (positive Homans' sign), redness, tenderness along superficial vein
Auscultation • Blood pressure	Pulse pressure may reach 100.	Varies, serial readings >170/95

G

Table continued on following page

G PHYSICAL ASSESSMENT: HEART AND PERIPHERAL CIRCULATION *(Continued)*
Geriatric Adaptations

Steps	Normal and/or Common Findings	Significant Deviations
• Heart sounds	Murmurs may be benign, due to stiffened valves. S_4 may be due to decreased left ventricle compliance.	Loud murmurs, pericardial friction rub, or arrhythmia
Palpation • Extremities	Pulses may be difficult to locate.	Absent or asymmetrical peripheral pulses
• Heart		Displaced PMI, thrill

R PHYSICAL ASSESSMENT: HEART AND PERIPHERAL CIRCULATION
Racial and Ethnic Adaptations

Steps	Normal and/or Common Findings	Significant Deviations
Inspection • *Extremities:* Note dependent edema, capillary refill.		Swelling, pale nail beds may indicate impending sickle cell crisis.
• Hair growth on feet, hands.	Smooth, hairless.	

PHYSICAL ASSESSMENT: HEART AND PERIPHERAL CIRCULATION *(Continued)*
Racial and Ethnic Adaptations

R

Steps	Normal and/or Common Findings	Significant Deviations
Auscultation • Heart sounds: Note rate, estimated heart size, murmurs		Tachycardia, cardiomegaly; systolic and/or diastolic murmurs, which may be indicative of impending sickle cell crisis.
• Blood pressure		Hypertension: Assess significance.

DIAGNOSTIC TESTS

May need to refer for:

- Cardiac catheterization
- Exercise stress test
- Chest x-ray
- Enzyme studies
- ECG
- CBC
- Triglycerides
- Cholesterol
- Echocardiogram

POSSIBLE NURSING DIAGNOSES

- Nutrition: altered, risk for more than body requirements
- Skin integrity, risk for impaired

- Cardiac output, decreased
- Tissue perfusion, altered
- Activity intolerance
- Fatigue
- Sensory-perceptual alterations
- Self-care deficit
- Role performance, altered
- Knowledge deficit

Clinical Alert

- **Report any unusual heart sounds.**
- **Report decreased circulation, venous insufficiency, or lower extremity ulcers.**
- **Report chest pain, dyspnea, or marked hypertension.**

SAMPLE DOCUMENTATION

BP 126/72, apical pulse 80, heart RRR, without murmurs, gallop, or rub. PMI at 5th ICS, MCL. Extremities symmetrically warm, pink, without edema or clubbing; peripheral pulses equally palpable +2 (carotid, radial, femoral, popliteal, posterior tibial, dorsalis pedis).

CLIENT AND FAMILY EDUCATION AND HOME HEALTH NOTES

Adult

- Discuss risk factors of heart disease.
- Explain principles of aerobic exercise and a low-fat, low-cholesterol diet in prevention of heart disease.

- Offer guidelines on stress management, including minimal use of caffeine, tobacco, and alcohol.
- Explain importance of unrestricted circulation and regular exercise. Instruct client to avoid sitting for prolonged periods, to elevate legs if necessary to sit for prolonged periods, to avoid tight clothing, especially socks and hosiery, and to avoid crossing the legs while sitting.
- Explain importance of having BP checked every 2 years or more often if elevated.
- Explain importance of having cholesterol checked every 5 years or more often if elevated.

Pediatric

- Explain to parents the importance of lifetime habits for good nutrition and exercise.
- Stress the need to include fats in the infant's and toddler's diet and the need to reduce fats in the child's diet.
- Discuss possible need for additional iron during infancy and adolescence.

Geriatric

- Instruct client to check with primary care provider (PCP) before starting an exercise program. Stop exercising when fatigued.
- Review medications and provide appropriate education. Explain the need to take medication as prescribed and the side effects to watch for.
- Teach about the importance of proper foot and skin care.
- Report any new shortness of breath, edema, and/or weight gain to physician.
- Monitor blood pressure and pulse rate as instructed by PCP.

- Teach client how to check blood pressure and pulse rate.

- Instruct the client to follow the regimen prescribed by his or her physician for any chronic diseases and to keep follow-up appointments.

- Provide information about programs to help people stop smoking.

- Instruct client to reduce saturated fat and sodium intake.

- Suggest that patient use stress reduction techniques such as deep breathing, progressive muscle relaxation, and guided imagery and reduce stressful stimuli from lifestyle.

ASSOCIATED COMMUNITY AGENCIES

- <u>American Heart Association:</u> Health promotion literature, CPR classes.

- <u>American Red Cross:</u> CPR classes

- <u>National Heart, Lung, and Blood Institute:</u> Information

CHAPTER 16

ABDOMEN

HISTORY

Adult

- Appetite
- Diet recall for the past 24 hours
- Dysphagia
- Weight gain or loss
- Use of alcohol, tobacco, caffeine: Duration, amount, frequency

- Bowel and/or bladder routines, problems
- <u>Indigestion, nausea, vomiting, diarrhea, pain, jaundice, flatulence, incontinence:</u> Causes, frequency, treatments
- <u>Pain:</u> Type, predisposing factors, time, relationship to eating
- Medications for bowel, indigestion
- History of hepatitis, ulcer, arthritis
- History of gastrointestinal diagnostic tests, surgery
- History of eating disorders
- Hepatitis vaccination

Pediatric

- Congenital anomalies
- Jaundice
- Pain or paroxysmal fussiness and intense crying
- Frequent spitting up
- Projectile vomiting
- Constipation, encopresis, crying while urinating, frequency of urinary tract infections (UTIs)
- Introduction to new foods
- Type and methods of feeding
- Parental concerns
- Milk intake
- Pica intake
- History of eating disorders
- Diarrhea, colic, failure to gain weight, weight loss

Geriatric

- Abdominal pain, specifying whether the pain is associated with eating
- Excessive belching, bloating, flatulence

- Changes in appetite (especially a decrease in appetite)
- Nausea, vomiting, diarrhea
- Hemorrhoids, changes in bowel habits
- Rectal bleeding, pain, or itching; hernia
- Bowel habits (constipation or incontinence), use of laxatives
- Change in appearance of stools (tarry, bloody, pencil-shaped)
- Nutritional assessment: Appetite and/or intake, any functional problems interfering with shopping for food or meal preparation, available external support for meal preparation, weight loss, albumin and total protein levels, financial barriers to good nutrition, swallowing difficulties, difficulty chewing, or mouth discomfort

Racial and Ethnic

- History of familial Mediterranean fever: Periodic peritonitis
- Travel experiences, especially exposure to parasites

EQUIPMENT

- Ink pen
- Stethoscope
- Tape measure
- Gloves

CLIENT PREPARATION

- Have client empty bladder.
- Have client lie on back with knees bent.

- Have parent hold child <3 years on lap if unable to lie on back.
- Place child's hand under yours during palpation if child is ticklish.

PHYSICAL ASSESSMENT: ABDOMEN

Adult

Steps	Normal and/or Common Findings	Significant Deviations
Inspection		
• *Shape:* Note symmetry, contour.	Flat, rounded	Protuberant scaphoid (Fig. 16–1), asymmetry, masses
• Check color.	Same as or lighter than other areas	Redness, cyanosis, jaundice, lesions (see Integumentary System)
• *Surface:* Note motion (respiratory, digestive).		Circulatory pulsations Dilated veins
Auscultation		
• Lightly place warmed stethoscope (diaphragm) over diaphragm.		
• *Abdomen:* Note bowel sounds; pitch, volume, frequency in four quadrants (Fig. 16–2).	Bowel sounds, 5–35/min	Absent bowel sounds (after 5 minutes' continuous listening), absence of borborygmus
• Assess aortic, renal, femoral, arteries.	No vascular sounds	Bruits, hums, rubs

Table continued on page 233

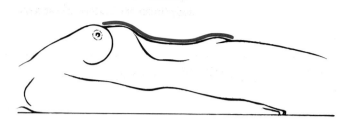

FIGURE 16–1
Scaphoid abdomen.

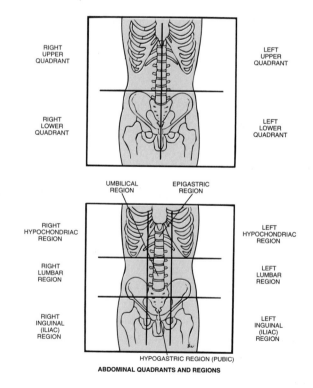

RIGHT
UPPER
QUADRANT

LEFT
UPPER
QUADRANT

RIGHT
LOWER
QUADRANT

LEFT
LOWER
QUADRANT

UMBILICAL
REGION

EPIGASTRIC
REGION

RIGHT
HYPOCHONDRIAC
REGION

LEFT
HYPOCHONDRIAC
REGION

RIGHT
LUMBAR
REGION

LEFT
LUMBAR
REGION

RIGHT
INGUINAL
(ILIAC)
REGION

LEFT
INGUINAL
(ILIAC)
REGION

HYPOGASTRIC REGION (PUBIC)

ABDOMINAL QUADRANTS AND REGIONS

FIGURE 16–2
Abdominal quadrants and regions. (*Source:* Adapted from Taber's, 1997, ed 18, p 3–4, with permission.)

PHYSICAL ASSESSMENT: ABDOMEN

A

(Continued)
Adult

Steps	Normal and/or Common Findings	Significant Deviations
Percussion		
• *Four quadrants:* Note percussion sounds (see Table 4–2).	Tympany, dullness	
• *Liver:* Note size. On right MCL, percuss upward from below umbilicus to dullness (lower border). Mark with pen at dullness. Move up to lung resonance and percuss downward in MCL to dullness (upper border of liver). Mark at dullness and measure (Fig. 16–3).	6–12 cm	Enlarged >12 cm or <6 cm
• *Liver scratch test:* Place stethoscope over liver; scratch skin surface lightly from middle of liver out toward periphery. Sound will diminish significantly when passing liver borders.		
• *Spleen:* Note size. Percuss on left side, distal to MCL (have client turn slightly to right side).	Should be between ribs 6 and 10	Enlarged

Table continued on following page

233

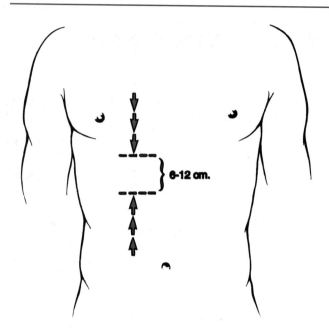

FIGURE 16–3
Percussion of liver.

PHYSICAL ASSESSMENT: ABDOMEN

(Continued)
Adult

Steps	Normal and/or Common Findings	Significant Deviations
Palpation Use the palmar surface of extended fingers.		
• *Abdominal wall:* Palpate lightly.	No tenderness, pain, masses	Tenderness, rigidity, nodules

PHYSICAL ASSESSMENT: ABDOMEN

A

(Continued)
Adult

Steps	Normal and/or Common Findings	Significant Deviations
• *Abdominal wall:* Palpate deeply (Fig. 16–4). Check four quadrants (see Fig. 16–2).		Tenderness, masses, bulges
• *Note organs:* Liver, spleen, kidneys.		
• *Aorta.*	Palpable in midline	Prominent lateral pulsation

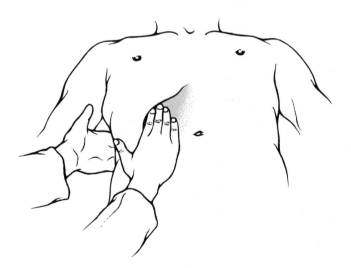

FIGURE 16–4
Palpation of liver.

P

PHYSICAL ASSESSMENT: ABDOMEN
Pediatric Adaptations
Neonate

Steps	Normal and/or Common Findings	Significant Deviations
Inspection • Shape of abdomen	Flat immediately following birth, then prominent and protuberant	Scaphoid abdomen in neonate may indicate diaphragmatic hernia Loose, wrinkled skin
• Umbilical cord	Presence of two umbilical arteries, thick white or cream-colored walls, and one vein	One umbilical artery Gastroschisis

P

PHYSICAL ASSESSMENT: ABDOMEN
Pediatric Adaptations
Infant

Steps	Normal and/or Common Findings	Significant Deviations
Inspection • Shape of abdomen.	Protuberant because of the underdeveloped musculature.	Umbilical or ventral herniations: diastasis recti; weakness of the musculature
• Motion.		Visible reverse peristalsis
• *Umbilical stump:* Note color, odor.	Stump falls off 10–15 days after birth.	Signs of infection; foul odor
Auscultation • Bowel sounds.	Listen every 10–30 seconds.	Absent (after 5 minutes' continuous listening), hyperactive

PHYSICAL ASSESSMENT: ABDOMEN

Ρ

(Continued)
Pediatric Adaptations
Infant

Steps	Normal and/or Common Findings	Significant Deviations
Palpation		
• Have infant supine; place folded blanket under infant's knees and hips to elevate feet and relax abdominal muscles. Because infants have limited verbal ability, observe infant for facial cues indicating discomfort.		
• Liver.	1–2 cm below right costal margin (RCM).	Enlarged
• Spleen tip.		Tenderness, mass, difficult to assess
• Bladder.		
• Descending colon.		
Percussion		
• Bladder.	May reach level of umbilicus at times. Children have more tympany than adults because of presence of more air in intestines.	

P

PHYSICAL ASSESSMENT: ABDOMEN
Pediatric Adaptations
  Child

Steps	Normal and/or Common Findings	Significant Deviations
Inspection • Assess shape of abdomen.	Abdomen should be protuberant when child is standing, flat when lying supine.	Distention Distended veins
• *Abdomen:* Note pulsations.		Marked aortic pulsation
Palpation • Place child's hand under yours to prevent tickling.		Child keeps knees drawn up, abdominal pain, splinting abdomen
• Assess liver edge.	Should be less than 3 cm below costal margin.	Enlarged liver
• Check bladder.	May be palpated just above the symphysis pubis in the preschooler.	
• Check spleen tip.	1–2 cm: Below LCM.	Enlarged spleen
• Assess lower poles of both kidneys.	Rarely palpable.	

G

PHYSICAL ASSESSMENT: ABDOMEN
Geriatric Adaptations

Steps	Normal and/or Common Findings	Significant Deviations
Inspection • Contour	Sagging, rounded because of loss of muscle tone and an increase in fat deposits	Marked distention or concavity

PHYSICAL ASSESSMENT: ABDOMEN

Geriatric Adaptations *(Continued)*

Steps	Normal and/or Common Findings	Significant Deviations
Auscultation • Assess bowel sounds.	Diminished peristalsis Hyperactive with large doses of laxatives	Absent after listening for 5 minutes
Palpation • (Deeper and firmer palpation may be required to elicit pain or rebound tenderness.)		
• *Liver:* Note size.	May be decreased, but may extend 2–3 cm below right costal margin because of enlarged lung fields	Markedly enlarged
• Check aorta.	May be dilated	Bruits

PHYSICAL ASSESSMENT: ABDOMEN

Racial and Ethnic Adaptations

Steps	Normal and/or Common Findings	Significant Deviations
Palpation • Note organ size.		Hepatomegaly, hyposplenism, or splenomegaly (sickle cell disease indications)

239

DIAGNOSTIC TESTS

May need to refer for:

- CBC
- Bilirubin
- Electrolytes
- Barium enema
- Stool guaiac
- Hepatic panel (liver enzymes)
- Endogastroduodenoscopy, colonoscopy, flexible sigmoidoscopy
- Abdominal ultrasound or CT scan

POSSIBLE NURSING DIAGNOSES

- Constipation, perceived or risk of
- Diarrhea
- Urinary elimination, altered
- Fluid volume, risk for deficit
- Nutrition: altered, less than or more than body requirements
- Sleep pattern disturbance

Clinical Alert

- **Absence of bowel sounds**
- **Palpable masses**
- **Enlarged spleen, liver**
- **Acute abdominal pain, nausea, or vomiting**
- **Changes in bowel habits or blood in stool**
- **Difficulty swallowing**
- **Dyspepsia**

SAMPLE DOCUMENTATION

Adult
- Abdomen smooth, rounded, nontender. Bowel sounds active in all quadrants. Liver size approximately 10 cm at MCL, not palpable. No organomegaly or masses palpated. No visible aortic pulsation and no bruits auscultated.

Child
- Pot-bellied appearance of abdomen. Soft. Bowel sounds present in all four quadrants. No hepatomegaly, splenomegaly, masses, or tenderness.

CLIENT AND FAMILY EDUCATION AND HOME HEALTH NOTES

Adult

- Explain the dynamics of a balanced diet in terms of calories, height, and activity. One formula, for example, that expresses the interrelationships among these factors is as follows: Ideal weight × 13-15-20 activity factor. Another useful formula to give to clients is the following: ≤30 percent fats (10 percent each: saturated, monounsaturated, polyunsaturated); cholesterol <300 mg daily; 12 percent protein; 48 percent carbohydrates; ≤10 percent refined sugar; and ≤5 g of salt daily.

- Review with the client the Food Guide Pyramid (App. Q).

- Review with the client the height and weight tables (App. R).

- Assess the client for physical signs of malnutrition and deficiency state as listed in Appendix S.

- To calculate the number of calories one can consume and lose weight, use the following formula. For women, multiply current weight by 10; for men multiply current weight by 12 (Edelman and Mandle, 1994).

- For a diet to be ≤30 percent fat, the calories from fat should not exceed*:

24-h Caloric Intake	Total Fat per Day	Saturated Fat
1600	≤53	<18
2200	≤73	<24
2800	≤93	<31

*Source: Adapted from Edelman, CL, and Mandle, CL: Health Promotion Throughout the Lifespan. Mosby–Year Book, St Louis, 1998, ed 4, p. 249. With permission.

- Assess client's salt intake. Be aware of hidden salt in canned goods and processed foods.
- Instruct client in how to read nutrition labels.

Pediatric

- Explain goals of basic nutrition to parents.
- Explain introduction of foods to infant:
  - <u>0 to 4 months:</u> Breast milk or formula only.
  - <u>4 months:</u> Breast milk or formula. Cereal made with breast milk or formula should be fed with spoon. Begin with 1 teaspoon twice daily; increase to 4 tablespoons twice daily.
  - <u>4½ to 5 months:</u> Add vegetables one at a time. Give for 1 week before starting another. Begin with 1 teaspoon; increase to 3 tablespoons twice daily.
  - <u>5 months:</u> Add fruits one at a time, in same way you introduced vegetables.
  - <u>6 to 8 months:</u> Add meats, one meat at a time, for a week as you introduced vegetables and fruits. Add beef last. Add fruit juice diluted with half water.
  - Continue to give formula or breast milk for 1 year, then whole milk until age 2. After 2 years give 2% milk.
- Encourage parents to offer a wide variety of nutritious foods and to avoid offering foods containing empty calories such as soft drinks, candy, and pastries.
- Explain toddler-preschool eating patterns, that is, food jags or strong preference for only a few foods. Teach parents to assess diet over several days rather than over one meal.

- Discuss the need for fat in the infant's and toddler's diet.

- Explain hazards of choking when toddler eats hot dogs or hard candy or chews on toys or balloons.

Geriatric (See also App. T)

- Teach techniques to prevent constipation:

  - Participate in regular exercise.

  - Drink at least 1500 to 2000 mL of fluid per day unless contraindicated by other health problems such as congestive heart disease, SIADH, or renal disease.

  - The following types of drugs may contribute to constipation: antihistamines, aspirin, antacids with aluminum or calcium, antiparkinsonism drugs, diuretics, tranquilizers, and hypnotics.

  - Reduce or eliminate use of laxatives because they can be harmful and habit forming.

  - Eat foods high in fiber, such as fresh fruits and vegetables and whole grains. Eat foods low in fat and refined sugar.

  - It is not necessary to have a bowel movement every day. Individuals have different patterns for elimination. If a person is not having problems with painful movements or hard stools and the frequency of movements is only once every 4 days or more, then the person is probably not constipated.

- Try to develop a regular schedule for bowel elimination, such as in the morning after breakfast.

- Respond promptly to the urge to defecate.

- Provide the following information to clients with fecal incontinence:

- It is important to seek help and receive a comprehensive workup to determine the etiology.
- Follow the same recommendations for fecal incontinence as those given above for constipation.
- If fecal impaction or long-term constipation is the problem, initiate the above recommendations following removal of the impaction.
- Establish a consistent toileting program and establish a routine time.
- Instruct client on pelvic muscle exercises.
- Provide frequent reminders of the location of the restroom if the client is cognitively impaired or in an unfamiliar environment.
- Teach client to be meticulous in skin care, use of absorbent products or external collection devices, and use of moisture barrier creams and to frequently assess the condition of the skin.

Racial and Ethnic

- Teach variations in preparation of health foods preferred in culture (e.g., boiled instead of fried, spices added to foods instead of salt).
- If lactose-intolerant (common in many Asians, African-Americans, Jews, and Mexican-Americans), suggest purchase of lactose-free milk or substitute other foods containing calcium such as yogurt.

ASSOCIATED COMMUNITY AGENCIES

- Assess the need for and refer as appropriate to:
  - <u>Food Stamp program:</u> Serves all ages.
  - <u>Supplemental Nutrition Program for Women, Infants, and Children (WIC):</u> Serves pregnant and

245

breast-feeding women and children up to the age of 5

- <u>Reduced price and free lunches, school breakfast program:</u> For school age children
- <u>Congregate meal sites:</u> Persons age 60 and older
- <u>Meals on Wheels:</u> Meals brought to home if no one in home is able to prepare
- <u>Food pantries:</u> At local churches or community centers (Contact United Way for information.)

- Ostomy clubs.
- National Digestive Diseases Clearinghouse
- Celiac Sprue Association
- Crohn's and Colitis Foundation of America

CHAPTER 17

MUSCULOSKELETAL SYSTEM

HISTORY

Adult

- Client's age
- Last menstrual period or years since menopause
- Weight
- Height, loss of height
- Tobacco use
- Ability to care for self, functional abilities
- Exercise patterns, equipment; athletic injuries
- Knowledge and use of good body mechanics, safety precautions
- <u>Muscular complaints:</u> Limitation of movement, weakness, tremor, tic, paralysis, clumsiness
- Assess dietary calcium, vitamin D, protein intake

- History of joint pain, swelling, heat, arthritis, bone injury (see App. U)
- <u>Skeletal complaints:</u> Difficulty with gait, limping, numbness, pain with movement, crepitus
- Joint, bone, muscle trauma
- Use of hormone replacement therapy
- <u>Medications:</u> Anti-inflammatory agents, aspirin
- Self or family history of osteoporosis, arthritis, fractures, muscle disease, tuberculosis, genetic or congenital disorders, cancer, scoliosis
- Orthopedic surgeries
- Employment

Pediatric
Infant

- Birth injuries, macrosomia
- Alignment of hips, knees, ankles
- Trauma
- Developmental milestones

Children

- Participation in sports, outdoor activities
- Frequent contact or high-impact fractures, limping, complaints of aches or pain in joints, other trauma

Geriatric

- Stiffness, backache
- History of falls, tremors, spontaneous fractures, fall-related fractures, stumbling
- <u>Weakness or pain with muscle use:</u> Location; weakness and activity altered
- Problems with manual dexterity

- Deformity or coordination difficulties
- Problems with shoes
- Restless legs; transient paresthesia
- <u>Alterations in gait:</u> Weakness, balance problems, difficulty with steps, fear of falling
- <u>Use of assistive devices:</u> Walker, cane, grab bars, elevated toilet seat, wheelchair
- Joint swelling, pain, redness, heat, deformity, stiffness: Pronounced at certain times of day/night, or associated with or following activity or inactivity
- <u>Limited movement:</u> Specify.
- Crepitation
- Able to carry out ADLs and IADLs. If not, who is available for assistance?

EQUIPMENT

- Tape measure
- Goniometer

CLIENT PREPARATION

- Sitting
- Supine
- Standing (observation of balance)
- Walking (observation of gait)
- Observation of child while playing

PHYSICAL ASSESSMENT: MUSCULOSKELETAL SYSTEM
Adult

A

Steps	Normal and/or Common Findings	Significant Deviations
Inspection		
• *Posture:* Note symmetry, erectness.	Erect, flexible, mobile, slumped, rounded shoulders	Spinal curvatures (Fig. 17–1) Legs of uneven length
• *Major muscle groups:* Note symmetry.	Atrophy, mild hypertrophy, bilateral symmetry	Marked or unexplained hypertrophy, asymmetry Marked or unexplained atrophy
• *Joints:* Note color. Observe neck, shoulder, elbow, wrist, hip, knee, ankle, foot (Figs. 17–2 through 17–5).	Full ROM	Edema, redness, heat, limitation in motion, deformities
• *Spine:* Have client bend at waist.	Full ROM	Curvature Kyphosis (see Fig. 17–1) Scoliosis Lordosis
Palpation		
• *Joints:* Note mobility, ROM, symmetry, temperature.	Full active and passive ROM	Tenderness, warmth, **edema**, **stiffness**, instability
• *Muscles:* Note tone and strength by having client resist pressure. Compare bilaterally.	Firm, tense on movement Strength 3+ to 4+	Soft, flabby Weakness 1+

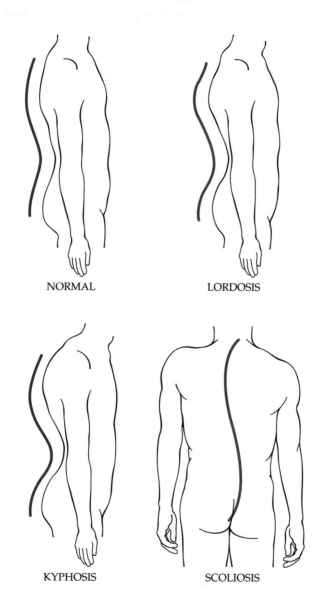

FIGURE 17–1
Normal and abnormal spinal curves.

NORMAL

LORDOSIS

KYPHOSIS

SCOLIOSIS

250

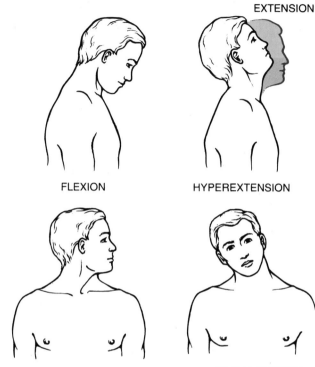

FLEXION

EXTENSION

HYPEREXTENSION

ROTATION

LATERAL FLEXION

FIGURE 17–2
Range of motion of neck.

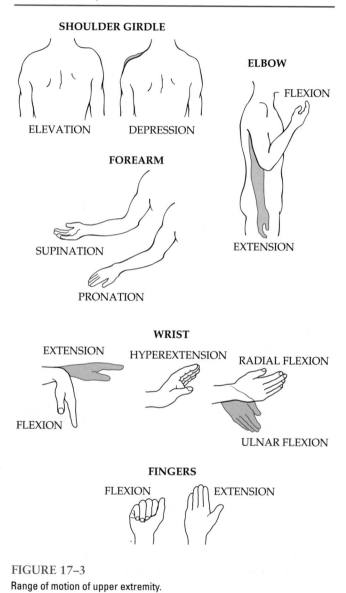

FIGURE 17–3

Range of motion of upper extremity.

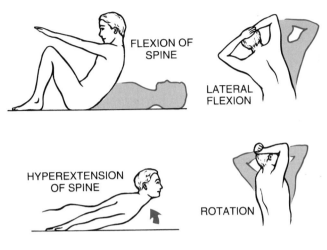

FIGURE 17–4

Range of motion of trunk.

PHYSICAL ASSESSMENT: MUSCULOSKELETAL SYSTEM

Pediatric Adaptations
  Infant

Steps	Normal and/or Common Findings	Significant Deviations
Inspection		
• Muscle tone	Isotonic	Decreased muscle tone Hypertonic Scissoring
• *Feet, legs:* Note tibial torsion and/or metatarsus adductus; if present, use gentle pressure in	Tibial torsion (should resolve after 6 months of age), flatfeet	Polydactyly or syndactyly Inability to straighten foot Clubfoot

Table continued on page 255

253

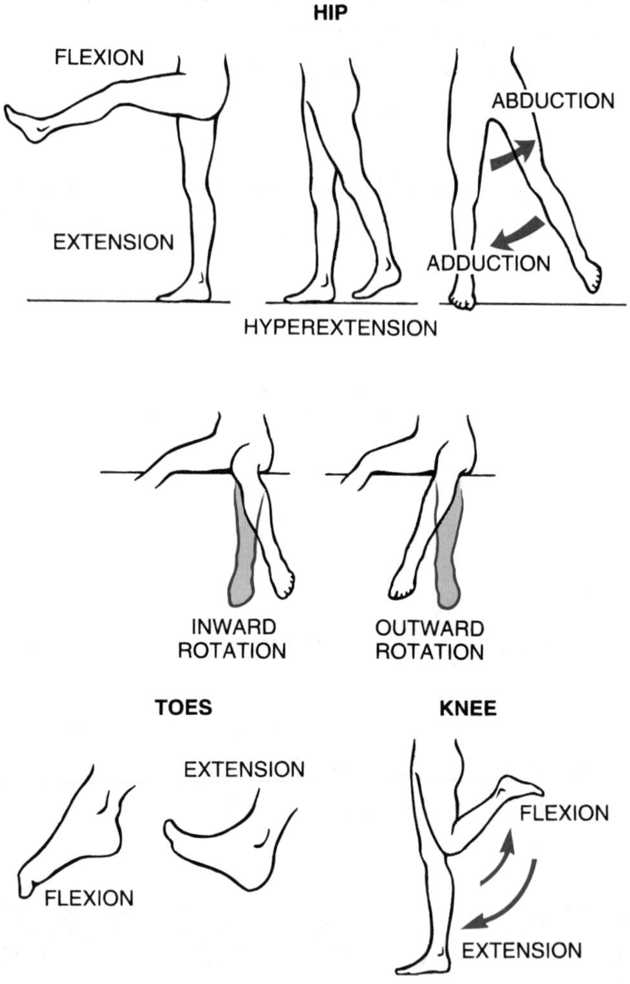

FIGURE 17–5

Range of motion of lower extremity.

PHYSICAL ASSESSMENT: MUSCULOSKELETAL SYSTEM *(Continued)*

Pediatric Adaptations
Infant

Steps	Normal and/or Common Findings	Significant Deviations
attempt to straighten foot.		
Palpation		
• Clavicles.	Intact	Fractures or absent
• Hips.	Equal gluteal folds, equal movement	Ortolani's sign (dislocation) (Fig. 17–6) Barlow's sign Unequal gluteal folds, limited ROM
• Spine.	Intact, smooth	Defects in vertebral column, dimples, or hair tufts
• ROM.	Full in all joints but may resist	
• *Muscles:* Note bilateral strength.	May elicit Moro response	Hypertonicity, flaccidity, unilateral weakness

PHYSICAL ASSESSMENT: MUSCULOSKELETAL SYSTEM

Pediatric Adaptations
Child

Steps	Normal and/or Common Findings	Significant Deviations
Inspection		
• Legs	Genu varum (bow-leg) and metatarsus adductus (normal to age 2)	Asymmetry Toeing in

Table continued on page 256

FIGURE 17–6

Hip dislocation in infant: Step 1: Flex infant's hips and knees. Place middle finger over greater trochanter. Step 2: Barlow-Ortolani maneuver—Abduct and adduct the thigh while in flexed position, feeling for a click or popping at greater trochanter.

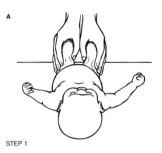

STEP 1

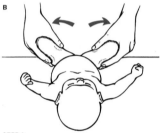

STEP 2

P

PHYSICAL ASSESSMENT: MUSCULOSKELETAL SYSTEM *(Continued)*

Pediatric Adaptations
Child

Steps	Normal and/or Common Findings	Significant Deviations
• Knees	Genu valgum (knock-knee) (from ages 2–10)	More than 2½ in between malleolus when knees are touching
• Spine	Increased lumbar curvature in toddlers	Scoliosis

PHYSICAL ASSESSMENT: MUSCULOSKELETAL SYSTEM

G

Geriatric Adaptations

Steps	Normal and/or Common Findings	Significant Deviations
Inspection		
(Client sitting)		
• Spine	Mild kyphosis	Severe kyphosis, scoliosis
• Joints of fingers, hands, wrists, shoulders, elbows, knees, ankles, toes	Limitation in normal ROM, instability	Swelling, nodules, heat, redness, crepitus, deformities (Fig. 17–7) Varus deformity (bowlegs) Valgus deformity (knock-knees)
• Muscles	Decreased muscle mass	Gross atrophy
• Feet	Corns, calluses, hammertoes, bunions	Joint swelling, redness
Test		
(Client standing)		
• *Spine:* Note ROM, symmetry, posture.	Abnormal curvature, especially kyphosis; slowed movement, diminished sense of balance; diminished muscle mass and strength bilaterally	Severe kyphosis, lordosis, scoliosis
Test		
(Client sitting)		
• *ROM:* Check neck, fingers, hands, wrists, shoulders, elbows.	Diminished joint flexibility bilaterally	ROM significantly impaired, affecting functional ability, marked pain

Table continued on page 259

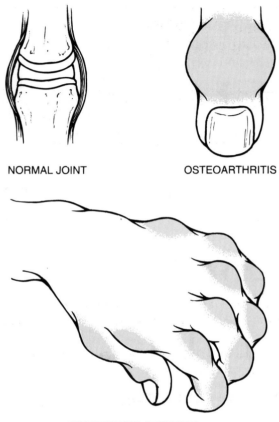

NORMAL JOINT　　　　OSTEOARTHRITIS

RHEUMATOID ARTHRITIS

FIGURE 17–7
Normal joint and deformities.

PHYSICAL ASSESSMENT: MUSCULOSKELETAL SYSTEM *(Continued)*

G

Geriatric Adaptations

Steps	Normal and/or Common Findings	Significant Deviations
• *ROM:* Check ankles, feet, knees, hips.	Diminished joint flexibility bilaterally	Joint swelling and redness
Palpation • Joint range of motion		Crepitus, tenderness

DIAGNOSTIC TESTS

May need to refer for:

- Bone densitometry to detect osteoporosis
- Blood tests for rheumatoid factor, calcium, and uric acid
- X-rays to detect compression fractures or other bone or joint abnormalities.

POSSIBLE NURSING DIAGNOSES

- Injury, risk for
- Mobility, impaired physical
- Sleep pattern disturbance
- Protection, altered
- Activity intolerance, risk for
- Fatigue
- Self-care deficit, toileting
- Pain, chronic

- Disuse syndrome, risk for
- Social isolation

Clinical Alert

- **Protect older clients from falling.**
- **Prevent contractures by exercise and ROM activities.**
- **Refer if there is sudden joint pain, swelling, erythema or ROM limitation, sudden muscle weakness, or new back pain.**

SAMPLE DOCUMENTATION

Adult

- Posture relaxed, erect; no lordosis, kyphosis, scoliosis visible. Joints mobile, nontender; full ROM demonstrated in every joint without pain or limitation. Muscle strength and size equal bilaterally. Gait smooth and steady.

Infant

- Extremities symmetrical, isotonic. Hips stable bilaterally. Spine straight, no tufts or dimples. Forefeet in varus position. Full passive range of motion.

Child

- Extremities symmetrical, isotonic. Full ROM in all four extremities. No scoliosis.

CLIENT AND FAMILY EDUCATION AND HOME HEALTH NOTES

Adult

- Instruct client to maintain muscle strength and joint flexibility through exercise.
- Teach appropriate exercise techniques.
- Teach risk factors associated with osteoporosis (sedentary lifestyle, poor dietary calcium, female, small bones, low weight, white, fair skin, smoking, heavy alcohol use). Encourage prevention beginning in youth, extending through lifetime.
- Teach safety risks associated with falls in home, such as loose rugs, poor lighting, uneven surfaces, wet surfaces (tub, bathroom floor).
- Instruct client to have a physical exam before beginning exercise program.
  - Exercise at least 20 minutes three times per week.
  - Before exercise, stretch and warm up.
  - During exercise, maintain heart rate of between 60 and 85 percent of capacity. Calculate this by subtracting your age from 220. Multiply this number by 0.60 to find the lower range and by 0.85 to obtain the higher range.
  - Cool down with stretching and milder exercise.

Pediatric

- Encourage physical fitness early with regular exercise.
- See Adult notes (above). Teach parents and adolescents about prevention of osteoporosis as well as maintenance of mobility.
- Teach safety precautions for the home.

261

- Instruct in use of protective devices when rollerblading and biking.

Geriatric

- Teach proper diet and exercise to reduce progression of osteoporosis.

- Teach about new methods to diagnose, treat, and reverse osteoporosis.

- Teach client how to manage chronic pain with prescribed medications and other modalities as appropriate (TENS unit, individualized exercise program, appropriate rest periods, articular rest, heat or cold therapy, paraffin baths for hands, splints or other assistive devices, weight loss, hydrotherapy and/or water exercises, surgical intervention.

- Teach client how to use assistive devices correctly.

- Teach client to avoid immobility.

- Teach safety measures to prevent falls:

  - Install nonslip mats and/or stick-ons in tubs and showers.

  - Use adequate lighting devices such as nonglare surfaces and night lights near stairs and/or stairwells.

  - Remove hazards such as throw rugs, electrical cords, loose carpet edges, clutter, and furniture from traffic pathways.

  - Hold onto rails along stairways for stabilization and support.

  - Ambulate with eyes facing ahead so you can scan the environment for any safety hazards.

  - Place grab bars near the toilet and tub.

  - Wear footwear with nonskid soles.

  - Ambulate carefully, and do not rush.

- Rise from a sitting position to a standing position very slowly to prevent orthostatic hypotension.
- Use emergency alert systems if they are available to you.

- If a client is being seen in the home, assess and document his or her homebound status on each visit.

- When clients have decreased mobility:
  - Observe ambulation.
  - Instruct in use of assistive devices.
  - If walker or wheelchair is to be used, check width of hallways and doorways for maneuverability.
  - Check proximity of bathroom to bedroom.
  - Adjust height of walker, commode, and/or cane prn.
  - Instruct in use of hospital bed and the importance of turning.
  - Client may need physical or occupational therapy evaluation and/or treatment to optimize function and safety.

℞ Racial and Ethnic

- Average Asian males are shorter than average white males.
- Average Asian females are shorter than average white females.
- Bones of average African-Americans are longer, narrower, and denser than those of other groups and are less apt to fracture.
- Bone density is the least in Asians.

ASSOCIATED COMMUNITY AGENCIES

- <u>Arthritis Foundation:</u> Arthritis self-help course, loans for equipment, public education
- <u>Transportation assistance:</u> American Red Cross
- <u>Home health agencies:</u> Homemaker assistance
- <u>Churches:</u> Help with building wheelchair ramps
- National Osteoporosis Foundation
- American Juvenile Arthritis Foundation
- Muscular Dystrophy Association
- National Scoliosis Foundation
- United Cerebral Palsy Association

CHAPTER 18

NEUROLOGIC SYSTEM

HISTORY

Adult

- Headaches
- Dizziness
- Visual disturbances
- Numbness, weakness, spasms
- Twitching, tremors
- Forgetfulness
- History of head injury, neurosurgery, nerve injury, syncope, hereditary disorders such as Tay-Sachs disease, Huntington's disease, muscular dystrophy
- Changes in senses of taste, smell, hearing
- Difficulty swallowing
- Speech difficulties
- Seizures

- Change in cognition, behavior, communication, memory
- Use of all medications: Antidepressants, anticonvulsants, antivertigo agents
- Use of alcohol or mood-altering medications
- Exposure to chemicals, pesticides
- Exposure to assault, for example, spousal abuse
- History of CVA in self or family

Pediatric

Infant

- Apgar score of infant (see App. G)
- Birth trauma; other trauma or infection
- Maternal alcohol or substance abuse
- Maternal or neonatal exposure to TORCH viruses (Toxoplasmosis, Other [Syphilis], Rubella, Cytomegalovirus, Herpes Simplex)
- Dietary intake for 24 hours
- Patterns of behavior and daily schedule
- Child-rearing practices, risk of abuse

Child

- Past head injuries, illnesses, fevers
- Attainment of developmental milestones: Exhibits head control, sitting, crawling, walking, speaking, fine motor control
- Change in behavior, personality, cognition, communication
- Daily schedule, preschool, games
- Fever, projectile vomiting
- Amount and type of television viewed
- Interactions

- Use of drugs
- Neck stiffness, high-pitched cry
- Child-rearing practices, risk of abuse

Geriatric

- Sensory disturbances: Paresthesia, hyperesthesia, diplopia
- Dizziness, faintness, spells, attacks, weakness, headaches
- Changes in gait, coordination, and balance; vertigo
- History of injuries or falls, particularly recent ones
- Mental status changes such as in mood, thinking process, or cognitive process
- Speech alterations
- How any symptoms affect ADL

EQUIPMENT

- Tuning fork
- Reflex hammer
- Cotton balls
- Familiar object: Coin, paper clip, button
- Sharp object

CLIENT PREPARATION

- Sitting
- Standing

PHYSICAL ASSESSMENT: NEUROLOGIC SYSTEM
Adult

Steps	Normal and/or Common Findings	Significant Deviations
	MOTOR/SENSORY	
Inspection		
• *Extremities:* Note coordination, gait, tremor.	Smooth motions, no tremor	Tremor; abnormal gaits such as shuffling
• *Large muscles:* Note symmetrical size, involuntary movements.	No involuntary movement Symmetrical (Muscles of dominant side may be slightly larger.)	
Test		
• *Romberg:* Have client stand with both eyes open, then closed, with arms at sides, feet together (20–30 seconds). Stand near client in case balance is lost	Minimal or no swaying	Drift, imbalance
Palpation		
• *Extremities:* Note touch perception (with cotton ball), vibratory perception (with tuning fork over bone). Distinguish between sharp and dull.	Equal perception of vibration	Absent or asymmetrical vibratory perception
• *Large muscles:* Note symmetrical strength against resistance.	Symmetrical	Unequal weakness

Table continued on following page

A

PHYSICAL ASSESSMENT: NEUROLOGIC SYSTEM *(Continued)*

Adult

REFLEXES		
Test • Biceps, triceps, brachioradialis, patellar knee jerk, Achilles, plantar (Figs. 18–1 through 18–3) using percussion hammer (Fig. 18–4).	+2	Diminished or increased responses

COGNITION AND/OR MENTAL STATUS		
(See Apps. D, E, and V.) **Test** • Orientation to person, place, time	Oriented × 3	Unable to orient self, setting, date
• *Memory:* Immediate, recent, remote, and old recall	Intact	Memory loss of significant immediate or recent events
• Affect and mood	Appropriate to setting and circumstance	Inappropriate emotional response
• Judgment and ability to abstract	Responds appropriately	Judgment impaired
• Thought content and process		Inappropriate

CRANIAL NERVES		
(Table 18–1.) **Test** (If not tested with above systems.)		

Table continued on page 272

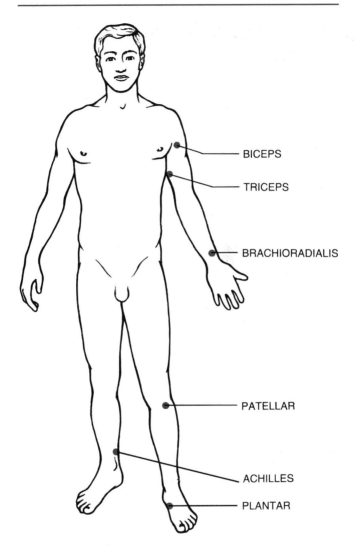

FIGURE 18–1
Reflexes.

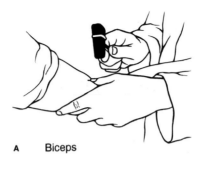

A Biceps

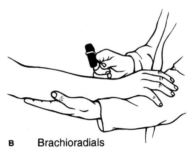

B Brachioradials

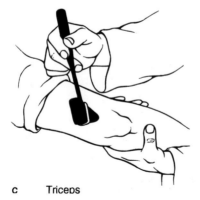

C Triceps

FIGURE 18–2

Eliciting deep tendon reflexes.

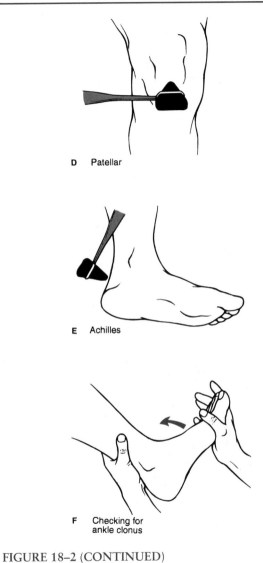

D Patellar

E Achilles

F Checking for ankle clonus

FIGURE 18–2 (CONTINUED)
Eliciting deep tendon reflexes.

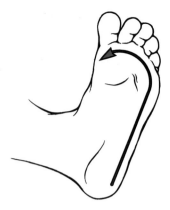

FIGURE 18–3
Eliciting the plantar reflex.

A

PHYSICAL ASSESSMENT: NEUROLOGIC SYSTEM *(Continued)*
Adult

Steps	Normal and/or Common Findings	Significant Deviations
CRANIAL NERVES		
• *CN I:* Ability to identify odors	Able to identify specific odors	Absence of sense of smell
• *CN II:* Visual acuity	Able to visualize all fields	
• *CN III:* Pupils, extraocular movements (EOMs)	Pupils constrict, eyes move through fields symmetrically	Asymmetrical pupillary response Nystagmus
• *CN IV:* Lid movements, EOMs	Even and symmetrical lid and eye movements	
• *CN V:* Facial sensation, muscle strength, corneal reflexes	Equal sensation and strength Blink symmetrical	Decreased or absent sensation; absent or asymmetrical blink
• *CN VI:* Lateral eye movements	Even eye movements	Absent or asymmetrical lateral eye movements

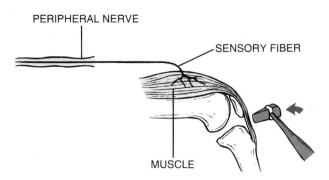

FIGURE 18–4

Use of percussion hammer to elicit reflex response.

PHYSICAL ASSESSMENT: NEUROLOGIC SYSTEM *(Continued)*
Adult

Steps	Normal and/or Common Findings	Significant Deviations
CRANIAL NERVES		
• *CN VII:* Facial muscle strength, taste	Symmetrical strength	Dropping lid Paralysis Decreased strength
• *CN VIII:* Hearing acuity, sound conduction	Equal acuity	Hearing loss
• *CN IX:* Taste, gag reflex	Voice smooth, gag reflex intact	Hoarseness; soft palate fails to rise or uvula deviates laterally
• *CN X:* Symmetry of uvula movement	Symmetrical rising of soft palate	Asymmetrical or diminished movement
• *CN XI:* Neck and shoulder strength	Symmetrical strength of trapezii and sternocleido-mastoid muscles	Weakness, unilateral or bilateral
• *CN XII:* Tongue-control, symmetry, strength	Even strength and motion of tongue	Fasciculations or deviation of tongue

TABLE 18-1 | CRANIAL NERVE FUNCTIONS AND ASSESSMENT METHODS

Cranial Nerve	Name	Type	Function	Assessment Methods
I	Olfactory	Sensory	Smell	Ask client to close eyes and identify different mild aromas, such as coffee, tobacco, vanilla, oil of cloves, peanut butter, orange, lemon, lime, chocolate.
II	Optic	Sensory	Vision and visual fields	Ask client to read Snellen chart, check visual fields by confrontation, and conduct an ophthalmoscopic examination.
III	Oculomotor	Motor	Extraocular movement (EOM); movement of sphincter of pupil; movement of ciliary muscles of lens	Assess six ocular movements and pupil reactions.
IV	Trochlear	Motor	EOM, specifically moves eyeball downward and laterally	Assess six ocular movements.

V	Trigeminal Ophthalmic branch	Sensory	Sensation of cornea, skin of face, and nasal mucosa	While client looks upward, lightly touch lateral sclera of eye to elicit blink reflex. To test light sensation, have client close eyes; then wipe a wisp of cotton over client's forehead and paranasal sinuses. To test deep sensation, alternately use blunt and sharp ends of a safety pin over same areas.
	Maxillary branch	Sensory	Sensation of skin of face and anterior oral cavity (tongue and teeth)	Assess skin sensation as for ophthalmic branch above.
	Mandibular branch	Motor and sensory	Muscles of mastication; sensation of skin of face	Ask client to clench teeth.
VI	Abducens	Motor	EOM; moves eyeball laterally	Assess six cardinal fields of gaze.
VII	Facial	Motor and sensory	Facial expression; taste (anterior two-thirds of tongue)	Ask client to smile, raise the eyebrows, frown, puff out cheeks, close eyes tightly. Ask client to identify various tastes placed on tip and sides of tongue: sugar (sweet), salt, lemon juice (sour), and quinine (bitter). Identify areas of taste.

Table continued on following page

TABLE 18–1 | CRANIAL NERVE FUNCTIONS AND ASSESSMENT METHODS *continued*

Cranial Nerve	Name	Type	Function	Assessment Methods
VIII	Auditory			
	Vestibular branch	Sensory	Equilibrium	Assessment methods are discussed with cerebellar functions (in next section).
	Cochlear branch	Sensory	Hearing	Assess client's ability to hear spoken word and vibrations of tuning fork.
IX	Glosso-pharyngeal	Motor and sensory	Swallowing ability and gag reflex, tongue movement, taste (posterior tongue)	Use tongue blade on posterior tongue while client says "ah" to elicit gag reflex. Apply tastes on posterior tongue for identification. Ask client to move tongue from side to side and up and down.
X	Vagus	Motor and sensory	Sensation of pharynx and larynx; swallowing; vocal cord movement	Assessed with CN IX; assess client's speech for hoarseness.

XI	Accessory	Motor	Head movement; shrugging of shoulders	Ask client to shrug shoulders against resistance from your hands and turn head to side against resistance from your hand. Repeat for other side.
XII	Hypoglossal	Motor	Protrusion of tongue	Ask client to protrude tongue at midline; then move it side to side.

Source: From Kozier, B, Erb, G, Blais, K, and Wilkinson, M: Fundamentals of Nursing, ed 5, p 545. Copyright 1998 by Addison-Wesley Longman. Reprinted by permission.

P

PHYSICAL ASSESSMENT: NEUROLOGIC SYSTEM

Pediatric Adaptations
Infant

Steps	Normal and/or Common Findings	Significant Deviations
Inspection		
• *Behavior:* Note alertness, positioning.	Irritability	Extreme irritability, tremors Brudzinski's or Kernig's sign
• *Crying:* Note pitch of cry.		High-pitched or cat's cry
• *Reflexes:* Moro, tonic neck, palmar and plantar grasp, Babinski, rooting, sucking.	All present in term newborn	Absence of reflexes
• Neck righting.	4–6 months old	
• Parachute.	8–9 months old	
• Muscle tone.	Firm recoil	Flaccid
• Observe for appropriate parent-infant interactions, stranger anxiety, parent's ability to soothe infant.	Separation anxiety greatest at 8–20 months	Inappropriate interactions and parental expectations; no separation anxiety
Palpation		
• Anterior and posterior fontanels.	Soft and flat	Bulging or markedly depressed
• *Touch:* Note response to touch in extremities in quiet-alert state.	Moves to touch	No response; exaggerated, jerky response; asymmetrical response
Test		
• *Hearing:* Note acoustic activity.	Responds by waking, or turning toward sound, or movement	No response to sounds

PHYSICAL ASSESSMENT: NEUROLOGIC SYSTEM (Continued)

P

Pediatric Adaptations
Infant

Steps	Normal and/or Common Findings	Significant Deviations
• Pupils.	PERRLA	Unequal pupillary response
Cranial Nerves		
• CN II, III, IV, VI	Infant should blink when light is shined in eyes	Absent, asymmetrical, or diminished response for each area tested for nerves I through XI
• CN V	Rooting and sucking reflex present	
• CN VII	Facial symmetry when crying, sucking, rooting	
• CN VIII	Blink or Moro reflex in response to clapping near side of head	
• *CN I and XI:* Cannot be tested in the infant.		
• *CN IX and X:* Similar to the adult.		

P

PHYSICAL ASSESSMENT: NEUROLOGIC SYSTEM

Pediatric Adaptations
Child

Steps	Normal and/or Common Findings	Significant Deviations
Inspection • Observe for appropriate parent-child interaction.	Increasing independence of child, decreasing control by parent.	Communication unclear; hostility; aggression; dependence.
• *Cerebral dominance:* Observe child while at play.	Preference for one hand or the other usually evident by age 3–4.	
Test • Speech	3-year-olds should be able to speak so that others can understand them 90% of the time.	Unclear speech.
Cranial Nerves • *CN II:* Snellen eye chart with pictures or E chart.		
• *CN III, IV, VI:* Use a new toy to test cardinal positions.		
• *CN V:* May offer child a cracker to test muscular strength of jaw.		
• Remaining CNs may be tested as for an adult.		
• Children who are 3–6 years old should be evaluated by the Denver II.		Abnormal results on the Denver II.

PHYSICAL ASSESSMENT: NEUROLOGIC SYSTEM

G

Geriatric Adaptations

Steps	Normal and/or Common Findings	Significant Deviations
Inspection • Face.		Tremors, asymmetry such as drooping of side of mouth, drooling from one side of mouth, asymmetrical wrinkling of forehead or subtle asymmetry of lines at corners of mouth
• Extremities.		Tremors, unilateral or symmetrical weakness, gait disturbances
• Emotional responses.		Labile, severely agitated, major behavioral changes
Test • *Mental acuity:* Note alterations.	Diminished memory for recent events	Marked change in mental status, poor judgment, limited attention span
• Heel-to-shin movement.	May not be able to perform	
• Gait.	Decreased balance, muscle tone, short steps, wide stance, slower gait	Gross unsteadiness, rigid arm movements, shuffling, marked impairment in balance and/or stability, extreme wide-based gait

Table continued on following page

G

PHYSICAL ASSESSMENT: NEUROLOGIC SYSTEM *(Continued)*
Geriatric Adaptations

Steps	Normal and/or Common Findings	Significant Deviations
• *Equilibrium:* Note: Do not ask geriatric clients to perform deep knee bends or hop in place on one foot. Most normal older people cannot do these maneuvers because of impaired position sense. Instead, observe client rising from chair.	Diminished; decreased vibratory sense in toes	Severe swaying, unable to maintain balance, **absent vibratory sensation in lower extremities**
Percussion		
• Deep tendon reflexes	May be diminished, especially the Achilles reflex	Hyperactive, absent, asymmetrical
Cranial Nerves		
• CN I	Sense of smell diminished	See significant deviations for the adult; sense of smell absent
• CN II	Presbyopia corrected with glasses.	Marked loss of vision Diminished peripheral vision Diminished color discrimination (especially blues, greens, and purples)
• CN III	Pupil size diminished, impaired accommodation, diminished upward gaze	Nonreactive pupils

PHYSICAL ASSESSMENT: NEUROLOGIC SYSTEM (Continued)
Geriatric Adaptations

Steps	Normal and/or Common Findings	Significant Deviations
• CN V	Sensory perception of pain; light touch may be diminished.	Absent
• CN VII	Diminished sense of taste	Absent
• CN VIII	Diminished hearing, especially of high-frequency sounds	Significant hearing loss
• CN IX and X	Diminished taste perception on posterior tongue	Absent
• CN XI	Diminished muscle strength	Marked muscle weakness, interferes with ADLs

DIAGNOSTIC TESTS

May need to refer for:

- CT scan
- MRI
- EEG
- Electrolytes, CBC, sedimentation rate, thyroid function tests, vitamin B_{12} and folate levels, RPR
- Spinal tap
- Neuropsychiatric testing

POSSIBLE NURSING DIAGNOSES

- Communication, impaired verbal
- Coping, individual, ineffective

- Mobility, impaired physical
- Swallowing, impaired
- Sensory-perceptual alterations (specify)
- Thought processes, altered
- Injury, risk for

Clinical Alert

- **Differentiate symptoms of dementia, delirium, and depression, and refer all cognitive and behavioral changes for diagnosis and treatment.**

SAMPLE DOCUMENTATION

Adult

- Gait, coordination smooth and steady. Extremities symmetrically strong; touch and vibratory sense intact. DTRs symmetrically +2 (biceps, triceps, brachioradialis, knee-jerk, ankle). Oriented × 3; Immediate, recent, and remote memory intact; thought, emotion grossly appropriate. Cranial nerves I–XII intact. Babinski negative laterally. Fine motor coordination intact. Balance intact. Romberg negative. Speech clear and follows directions without difficulty.

Infant

- Alert. Fontanelle soft and flat. Moro and palmar grasp reflexes present. Positive Babinski. Normocephalic. PERRLA.

Child

- Alert, cooperative. Oriented × 3. Cranial nerves II–VIII intact. Climbs stairs unassisted. Denver II scores normal. ~~PERRLA~~.

CLIENT AND FAMILY EDUCATION AND HOME HEALTH NOTES

Adult

- ~~P~~revent head injury with seat belts, helmets.
- ~~P~~revent motor vehicle accidents. Observe speed limits and do not drink and drive.
- ~~R~~ead labels of pesticides and chemicals, and observe precautions.
- ~~B~~e aware of available information and services to deter violence, practice stress management, and do not abuse drugs.

Pediatric

- Discuss developmentally appropriate infant stimulation activities.
- ~~P~~rotect infants and toddlers from traumatic falls.
- Teach parents and children use of seat belts, helmets, and car seats.
- Teach sports and recreation safety (e.g., use spotters for gymnastics, never swim alone, never dive in unknown waters, and observe cautions on toys, including age appropriateness).
- Teach parents how to avoid children's accidental ingestion of poisons, drugs, chemicals. All such products should be stored out of sight and reach, behind a locked door if possible.
- Instruct parents to keep syrup of ipecac on hand and to post poison control number on telephone.

C **Geriatric**

- Maintain activities that stimulate the mind.
- Have diminished vision and hearing assessed and treated.
- Maintain physical activities and exercise.
- Take care to avoid extreme heat and cold.
- Use assistive devices correctly, and follow safety precautions for the sensory impaired. Prevent falls.
- Seek medical help immediately if mental status or marked behavioral changes are noted.

ASSOCIATED COMMUNITY AGENCIES

- National Spinal Cord Injury Association
- Alzheimer's Disease and Related Disorders Association
- Local chapter of the Mental Health Association
- Epilepsy Foundation of America
- Spina Bifida Association of America

CHAPTER 19

MALE GENITOURINARY SYSTEM AND RECTUM

HISTORY

🗎 **Adult**

- Client's age
- Diet, use of alcohol
- Frequency, urgency, dysuria, nocturia
- Difficulty starting or stopping urinary stream
- Dribbling or weak stream

- Blood in urine; discharge
- Changes in bowel or bladder function
- Pain, lesions, or masses on penis, scrotum, inguinal area, anus
- Circumcised
- Back pain
- Contraceptive use
- Swelling of scrotum
- History of prostatitis, UTIs, pyelonephritis, cancer, diabetes, arthritis, cardiac or respiratory disease
- History of surgery, trauma, hernia
- Infertility
- Satisfied with sexual activity
- Impotence, difficulty getting or maintaining erection, difficulty with ejaculation
- Sexually transmitted diseases
- Self-examination techniques, frequency
- Sexual partner preference
- Risk factors for HIV, safer sex practices
- Hemorrhoids
- Rectal bleeding, blood in stools, pain
- Use of protective or supportive devices when exercising
- Travel history, areas with high incidences of parasitic infection
- Family history of colon or prostate cancer, rectal polyps

Pediatric

- Number of wet diapers per day
- Perianal itching
- Meconium ileus

- Chronic constipation, diarrhea, mucorrhea, steatorrhea
- Enuresis
- Encopresis
- UTIs
- Age of toilet training
- Congenital anomalies
- Hygiene practices: Circumcised, uncircumcised
- Scrotal swelling
- Mother's use of hormones during pregnancy
- Sexual activity (adolescent); knowledge level

Geriatric

- Duration and characteristics of urinary incontinence
- Frequency and amount of continent and incontinent voids
- Precipitants of incontinence
- Past treatments for urinary incontinence and its effects
- History of recurrent UTIs
- Other lower urinary tract symptoms: Frequency, urgency, dysuria, feeling of incomplete emptying or retention, straining to void, hesitancy in starting urine stream, weak urine stream, nocturia, hematuria, postvoid drip
- Use of condoms, catheters, briefs, or other protective products
- History of bowel habits: Constipation, fecal incontinence
- Fluid and dietary intake patterns
- Medications: Prescribed and over the counter

- Urethral discharge or burning
- Functional or cognitive deficits that interfere with sexual activity or continence
- Decline in frequency of or satisfaction with sexual activity
- Any treatment or surgery for prostate enlargement or a hernia
- Erectile dysfunction (difficulty achieving or maintaining an erection sufficient for intercourse) or difficulties in achieving an orgasm
- Difficulty retracting the foreskin
- Anal sphincter tone

EQUIPMENT

- Gloves
- Lubricant
- Thermometer (for neonates)
- Drapes
- Penlight

CLIENT PREPARATION

- Supine
- Standing
- Bending over
- Consider developmental age in discussing exam with child

A

PHYSICAL ASSESSMENT: MALE GENITOURINARY SYSTEM AND RECTUM
Adult

Steps	Normal and/or Common Findings	Significant Deviations
Inspection		
• *Hair:* Note distribution, foreign bodies.	Parasites	
• Skin of penis, scrotum, inguinal area.	Intact, smooth, wrinkled, rugae on scrotum	Lesions, rashes, nodules, edema, body lice
• *Penis:* Note prepuce, glans, foreskin, circumcision, position of urinary meatus (Table 19–1).	No lesions, discharge Foreskin easily retracted, if present Located at tip	Phimosis, chancre, warts, ulcers, discharge Displacement on dorsal or ventral side of penis
• Anus.	Hemorrhoids	Lesions, polyps, bleeding Very tender or painful
Palpation Use gloves.		
• Shaft of penis.	Slightly tender	Discharge from urinary meatus; nodules, masses, lesions
• *Testicles:* Note size.	Smooth, one side usually larger than other, left side lower than right, freely movable. Determine consistency—fluid-filled, gas, or solid material	Tenderness, nodules, ulcers, lesions, pain, enlarged
• Transluminate scrotum if mass other than testes.		

TABLE 19–1	STAGES OF SECONDARY CHARACTERIS- TICS: MALE GENITAL DEVELOPMENT
Development	**Characteristic**
A. Hair growth	1. None 2. Scant fine hair at the base of the penis 3. Darker and curlier hair 4. Adult type but less hair 5. Adult
B. Genital development	1. No change 2. Larger scrotum and testes, skin redder 3. Enlargement of penis 4. Further enlargement of penis, scrotal skin thickening 5. Adult

Source: Adapted from Tanner, JM: Growth at Adolescence, ed 2. Blackwell Scientific Publications, Oxford, England, 1962.

PHYSICAL ASSESSMENT: MALE GENITOURINARY SYSTEM AND RECTUM

(Continued)
Adult

Steps	Normal and/or Common Findings	Significant Deviations
• Inguinal, femoral area.	No masses, nodes	Hernias, enlarged nodes
• Anus and rectum.	Hemorrhoids	Inflammation, rashes, lesions, tenderness, induration Masses
• *Prostate:* With client leaning over table, gently insert gloved, lubricated index finger into rectum. Note size, consistency.	Smooth, rubbery; should be able to palpate only about 1 cm of gland; soft	Tenderness, nodules, masses; >1 cm protruding into rectum; firm, hard

P

PHYSICAL ASSESSMENT: MALE GENITOURINARY SYSTEM AND RECTUM

Pediatric Adaptations
Infant

Steps	Normal and/or Common Findings	Significant Deviations
Inspection		
• *Penis:* Note prepuce and glans.	Smooth, nontender, moist. Prepuce covers glans.	Redness, tenderness, swelling
• *Urethral meatus:* Note placement. Retract foreskin in uncircumcised males only enough to see urinary meatus. Do not break adhesions.	Centered at tip of penis.	Hypospadius (meatus on ventral surface) Epispadius (meatus on dorsal surface)
• Scrotum.	Well rugated	Absence of rugae or underdeveloped scrotum
• Anus.	Patent	Absent, occluded, signs of trauma
• Meconium.	Should pass within 24 hours of birth	Meconium ileus
Palpation		
• *Testicles:* To check for their presence in scrotum, position child cross-legged and sitting to prevent retraction of testes.	Both palpable	Either or both absent
• Inguinal canal	Intact	Herniations, bulges
• *Test:* If perianal itching, place tape against perianal folds. Examine with microscope.	No nematodes visible	Nematodes Pinworms

PHYSICAL ASSESSMENT: MALE GENITOURINARY SYSTEM AND RECTUM

P

(Continued)
Pediatric Adaptations
Infant

Steps	Normal and/or Common Findings	Significant Deviations
• *Test:* Anal patency can be checked in neonates by cautiously inserting a lubricated rectal thermometer if stools are not passed within first 24 hours of life.	Anus patent	Unable to insert thermometer

PHYSICAL ASSESSMENT: MALE GENITOURINARY SYSTEM AND RECTUM

G

Geriatric Adaptations

Steps	Normal and/or Common Findings	Significant Deviations
Inspection		
• *Pubic hair:* Note amount and distribution.	Diminished if not absent	
• *Penis:* Retract foreskin, if present, to examine head of penis. Note hygiene.	Decreased in size Many men > age 75 have not been circumcised.	Drainage, infection, lesions, nodules, tenderness, swelling of penis, inability to retract foreskin, painful retraction
• Scrotum.	Pendulous	Rashes, excoriation, lesions, edema, fewer rugae

Table continued on following page

G

PHYSICAL ASSESSMENT: MALE GENITOURINARY SYSTEM AND RECTUM

(Continued)

Geriatric Adaptations

Steps	Normal and/or Common Findings	Significant Deviations
Palpation		
• *Testes:* Note size.	Small, atrophied	Enlarged, nodular, fixed, tender
• Rectum.		Bleeding
• Prostate.	Enlarged prostate, relaxed rectal sphincter tone	Fecal impaction, grossly lax sphincter tone, hemorrhoids, masses
		Markedly enlarged, boggy or rubbery, hard and nodular, tender

DIAGNOSTIC TESTS

May need to refer for:

- Culture, if drainage is present
- Fecal swab for guaiac test
- Prostate-specific antigen (PSA), blood test, or prostate ultrasound or biopsy
- Urinalysis
- Urodynamic testing; comprehensive workup for urinary and/or fecal incontinence
- Sexual dysfunction workup

POSSIBLE NURSING DIAGNOSES

- Infection, risk for
- Constipation

- Nutrition: altered
- Fluid volume, risk for deficit
- Urinary elimination, altered
- Urinary retention
- Sexual dysfunction
- Sexuality patterns, altered
- Self-care deficit, bathing/hygiene
- Self-care deficit, toileting
- Rape-trauma syndrome

Clinical Alert

- **Maintain client's privacy, and reduce embarrassment as much as possible.**
- **Prevent trauma to hemorrhoids.**
- **Refer any complaints of dysuria, hematuria, difficulty voiding, penile lesions, discharge, or sexual dysfunction**

SAMPLE DOCUMENTATION

Adult

- Skin of genitalia smooth, dry, nontender. Circumcised penis without discharge or lesions. Testes smooth, not enlarged. No hernias palpated. Prostate border palpable; smooth, firm, nontender. Rectum without internal or external hemorrhoids or masses. Small amount of soft stool palpable in lower rectal vault and sphincter tone strong. Perianal area intact; sphincter tightens evenly.

295

Infant

- Penis uncircumcised. Foreskin retracts freely. Meatus at tip of penis. Testes descended bilaterally. Anus patent.

CLIENT AND FAMILY EDUCATION AND HOME HEALTH NOTES

Adult

- Instruct male clients to begin testicular self-examination (TSE) (Fig. 19–1) in their midteens.
- Explain prevention of sexually transmitted diseases by limiting activity to one, mutually monogamous, uninfected partner; if not possible, use condom with every exposure; emphasize risk of multiple partners.
- Instruct men to have rectal examination annually after age 40.

Pediatric

- Explain testicular examination.
- Discuss sexual development and activities as appropriate for age.
- Teach parents and child how to keep uncircumcised penis clean.
- Discuss with parents ways to teach child to prevent sexual abuse.

Geriatric

- Encourage intake of 2000 to 3000 mL of fluid daily unless clinically contraindicated.
- Teach patient to avoid micturition syncope in bathroom as it could result in a serious fall. Teach client to sit down to void.

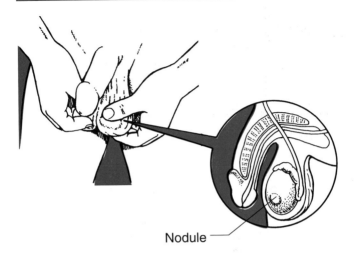

Nodule

FIGURE 19–1

Testicular self-examination. Instruct client to roll each testicle gently between thumb and fingers of both hands, feeling for lumps or nodules.

- Following a transurethral resection of prostate (TURP), it is important that the client understand that he will experience retrograde ejaculation.

- Sexual activity can continue well into a man's nineties or beyond, barring any major physical obstacles. Teach that it may take longer for an erection to occur, the erection may not be as firm as when he was younger, and it also may take more direct stimulation to achieve an erection. Ask physician about medications or devices if needed.

- If not circumcised, teach client to keep head of penis clean.

- Teach male and female clients to use water-soluble lubricant if needed during intercourse.

- Fecal and urinary incontinence are treatable conditions, but it is crucial that the client seek help from a health-care provider early. If the health-care provider does not respond to requests for testing and assistance with an incontinence problem, instruct client to seek help from a specialist, such as a urologist, a geriatrician, or an advanced practice nurse who specializes in such problems.

ASSOCIATED COMMUNITY AGENCIES

- National Association for Continence: Patient advocacy and education
- <u>National Kidney Foundation:</u> Local screening programs, education, and counseling
- <u>National Kidney and Urologic Diseases Information Clearinghouse:</u> Education
- Children's Organ Transplant Association
- Polycystic Kidney Disease Research Foundation

CHAPTER 20
FEMALE GENITOURINARY SYSTEM AND RECTUM

HISTORY

Adult
- Menstrual history
  - Age at menarche
  - Last menstrual period
  - Character, length, regularity of menses
  - <u>Dysmenorrhea:</u> Nature, severity, treatment
  - <u>Premenstrual changes:</u> Nature, severity, treatment

- Sexual history
  - Age of first coital experience
  - Number of different partners
  - Sexual partner preference
  - Satisfactions, problems
- Contraceptive history
  - Current and previous methods used
  - Current method: Satisfaction, consistency, questions or problems noted
- Obstetric history
  - Gravidity, parity: Term, preterm, living children
  - Abortions: Spontaneous, induced
  - Previous pregnancies: Complications with pregnancy, delivery, newborn
- Use of these products: Douche, sprays, deodorants, antiseptic soaps, talcum powder
- Dates of last Pap smear and pelvic examination
- History of vaginitis, cystitis, pyelonephritis, in utero exposure to DES, sexually transmitted diseases
- Recent change in any of the following: Bleeding, pain, vaginal discharge
- History of gynecologic/urologic surgeries
- History of sexual assault, incest; stage in crisis resolution
- Risk factors for HIV, safer sex practices
- Urinary function
  - Dysuria
  - Urinary urgency, frequency
  - Hematuria
  - Urinary incontinence
  - Infections: Chronic, related to coitus

Pediatrics

- Hygenic practices:
  - Use of bubble baths, irritating soaps, powders
  - Number of layers of clothing
  - Wearing cotton underpants
  - Cleansing perineal area front to back
- <u>Signs of sexual abuse:</u> Trauma, skin color changes in perineal area; history of bleeding, itching; inappropriate adultlike sexual knowledge, language, or behavior; sexually transmitted diseases

Geriatric

- Duration and characteristics of urinary incontinence
- Frequency and amount of continent and incontinent voids
- Precipitants of incontinence
- Past treatments for urinary incontinence and its effects
- History of recurrent urinary tract infections (UTIs)
- <u>Other lower urinary tract symptoms:</u> Frequency, urgency, dysuria, feeling of incomplete emptying or retention, straining to void, hesitancy, nocturia, hematuria
- Use of pads, briefs, or other protective products
- History of constipation
- Fluid and dietary intake patterns
- <u>Medications:</u> Prescribed and over the counter
- Urethral and/or vaginal discharge or burning
- Functional or cognitive deficits that interfere with sexual activity or continence; any adaptations made

- <u>Reproductive history:</u> Number of children, types of deliveries, complications
- <u>Menopausal history:</u> Date, difficulties, satisfactions
- Soreness, tenderness, dryness of vaginal wall
- Dyspareunia; decline in frequency of or enjoyment of sexual activity
- Pressure or heavy sensation in genital or pelvic area
- Vaginal bleeding after menopause
- Anal sphincter tone

EQUIPMENT

- Gown, drape
- New, clean glove
- Water-soluble lubricant
- Flexible floor lamp
- Pap smear equipment
- Speculum (may need pediatric size for both young women and older women who are no longer sexually active)
- Sterile cotton swabs/glass slide
- DNA probe kit for gonorrhea and chlamydia

CLIENT PREPARATION

- Have client empty bladder before examination.
- Drape fully in lithotomy position.
- Alternative positions may be necessary for women with disabilities.
- Offer mirror to explain findings to client.
- Warm speculum to body temperature.
- Place child in frog-leg position.

A

PHYSICAL ASSESSMENT: EXTERNAL STRUCTURES
Adult

Steps	Normal and/or Common Findings	Significant Deviations
Inspection		
• *Hair:* Note distribution, amount, foreign bodies.	Coarse, full, symmetrical	Uneven or unusually sparse Lice
• *Labia:* Note color, vascularity, moisture, symmetry, discharge, lesions, odor.	Pink to red; moist, symmetrical Scant to moderate white, nonodorous discharge	**Pale**, inflamed **Varicosities** **Dry** **Edema or swelling, especially unilaterally** **Dry, caked discharge** Copious, watery, thickened, or foul-smelling, white-yellow or green discharge, lesions
• *Clitoris:* Note size, color, lesions.	2 × 0.5 cm; same color as surrounding tissue	Atrophied or enlarged; reddened
• *Vaginal and urinary orifices:* Note color, lesions, moisture, size, bulging of vaginal wall.	Pink to red, moist, smooth; no lesions bulging	Reddened; lesions (ulcers, blisters, condyloma acuminata), **edematous irritated** Bulging of anterior or posterior vaginal wall on straining
• *Anus:* Note integrity.	Wrinkled, coarsened texture	Fissures, hemorrhoids (Fig. 20–1), lesions
Palpation		
• *Labia:* Note masses, tenderness, integrity.	Smooth, nontender, homogenous tissue	Nodules, painful to touch, **irregularities**

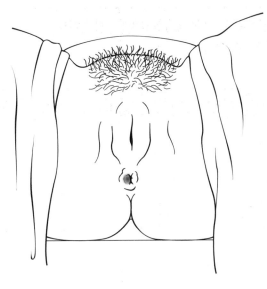

FIGURE 20–1

External hemorrhoid.

PHYSICAL ASSESSMENT: EXTERNAL STRUCTURES *(Continued)*
Adult

Steps	Normal and/or Common Findings	Significant Deviations
• *Skene glands:* Use one finger to press upward and later-ally and laterally in-side vagina, draw-ing finger toward outside of vagina. Observe for drain-age from gland.	No discharge Openings not visible	Discharge (culture) Openings visible

Table continued on following page

A

PHYSICAL ASSESSMENT: EXTERNAL STRUCTURES *(Continued)*
Adult

Steps	Normal and/or Common Findings	Significant Deviations
• Bartholin glands.	No tenderness or edema	Redness, tenderness, swelling of labia, especially unilaterally
• *Vaginal orifices:* Use thumb and forefinger; gently pinch around sides and perianal area. Note tenderness, masses.	No masses, nontender	Nodules, painful to touch
• With finger in vagina, ask client to tighten muscles and bear down. Note strength, bulges, urinary incontinence.	Tight muscles, no bulges, no incontinence	Bulging of anterior or posterior wall, urinary incontinence, protrusion of cervix

A

PHYSICAL ASSESSMENT: INTERNAL STRUCTURES
Adult

To insert vaginal speculum: Warm speculum with water. Insert two fingers into vagina and press down firmly; insert closed speculum at an angle over fingers, keeping blades at 45-degree downward angle. Rotate speculum back to horizontal level and gently open blades.

PHYSICAL ASSESSMENT: INTERNAL STRUCTURES (Continued)

Adult

Steps	Normal and/or Common Findings	Significant Deviations
Inspection		
• *Mucosa:* Note color, integrity, lesions, discharge.	Pink to red; smooth, moist, clear to white odorless discharge	Bright red or pale; lesions, fissures, inflamed areas, discharge
• *Cervix:* Note color, position, surface, discharge, os, lesions.	Evenly pink, midline, smooth surface or small, raised, light nabothian cysts Discharge odorless, clear to white; os small, round, or horizontal slit	Blue, reddened, pale Deviate laterally Patches of red or white tissue, friability increased Heavy, malodorous, yellow to green to gray discharge

PHYSICAL ASSESSMENT: OBTAINING PAP SMEARS

Adult

With speculum in place, obtain cells from cervical os, cervical border, and vaginal pool. Use spatula and cytobrush, and label slides with client's name and birth date before spraying with fixative. (To withdraw speculum: Close blades, rotate 45 degrees, gently remove, and avoid pinching.)

Steps	Normal and/or Common Findings	Significant Deviations
Palpation		
Insert gloved index and middle fingers into vagina and place nondominant		

Table continued on following page

A

PHYSICAL ASSESSMENT: OBTAINING PAP SMEARS *(Continued)*
Adult

Steps	Normal and/or Common Findings	Significant Deviations
hand on lower abdomen. Trap internal structures between your hands.		
• *Cervix:* Note consistency, surface, position, mobility, tenderness, patency of os.	Firm, smooth, midline, mobile to 2 cm, nontender, patent	Boggy, nodules, lateral deviations, fixed, painful with lateral movement, **strictures at os**
• *Uterus:* Note position, size, shape, mobility, tenderness, masses.	Midline; pear-shaped, 6–8 cm in length, slight AP mobility without tenderness	Lateral deviation, **unilateral or bilateral** masses, fixed, **tender** or painful to touch
• *Ovaries:* Note size, shape, tenderness, consistency, masses.	May not be palpable; approximately 3×2 cm, slightly tender, smooth, firm	Enlarged, nodular, **asymmetrical,** painful
Change gloves. Lubricate. Insert index finger into vagina, middle finger into rectum.		
• *Uterus:* Note shape, masses.	Smooth, uniform, no masses	Masses, irregular shape
• *Rectal wall:* Note masses, tenderness, tone. (Obtain stool specimen from gloved hand.)	Smooth, nontender, firm muscle tone	Nodules, masses, lesions **Tender** **Absent tone**

PHYSICAL ASSESSMENT: EXTERNAL AND INTERNAL STRUCTURES

Pediatric Adaptations
Infant

Steps	Normal and/or Common Findings	Significant Deviations
Inspection		
• *Discharge:* Note presence.	Absent or slight white discharge or blood in first week	
• *Labia:* Note size, position.	Edematous, slightly opened	Ambiguous genitalia
• *Vaginal opening:* Note presence.	Patent	Absence of vaginal opening
• Anus	Meconium passed in first 24 hours	No meconium in first 24 hours

PHYSICAL ASSESSMENT: EXTERNAL AND INTERNAL STRUCTURES

Pediatric Adaptations
Child

Steps	Normal and/or Common Findings	Significant Deviations
Inspection		
Note: complete gynecologic examinations, including Pap smear, should begin when individual becomes sexually active or at age 18–20.		

Table continued on following page

307

P

PHYSICAL ASSESSMENT: EXTERNAL AND INTERNAL STRUCTURES *(Continued)*

Pediatric Adaptations
Child

Steps	Normal and/or Common Findings	Significant Deviations
• Hair growth.	No hair; preadolescent Slight fine hair on labia majora; hair darker, thicker but finer texture and amount less than adult	Pubic hair before 9 years old
• *Genital region:* Note signs of sexual abuse.	No signs of abuse Hymenal tag	Scarring, lesions, red or darkened pigment, poor sphincter tone, vaginal odor (and other signs of infection), bleeding, pain, presence of STDs

G

PHYSICAL ASSESSMENT: EXTERNAL AND INTERNAL STRUCTURES

Geriatric Adaptations

Steps	Normal and/or Common Findings	Significant Deviations
Inspection		
• External genitalia	Atrophied; diminished fat pads; sparse, white hair	Masses, lesions, nodules, inflammation, gross asymmetry, erythema
• Mucosa	Pale, thin, friable	Tears, lesions, erythematous

PHYSICAL ASSESSMENT: EXTERNAL AND INTERNAL STRUCTURES *(Continued)*
Geriatric Adaptations

G

Steps	Normal and/or Common Findings	Significant Deviations
• Secretions, discharges	Scanty to absent	Colored, malodorous, or abundant discharges, **urinary incontinence**
• Uterus, ovaries	Nontender, atrophied, smaller; ovaries not palpable	Pain, asymmetry, enlarged, rectocele, cystocele, uterine prolapse

PHYSICAL ASSESSMENT: EXTERNAL STRUCTURES
Racial and Ethnic Adaptations

R

Steps	Normal and/or Common Findings	Significant Deviations
Inspection • Labia majora	Darker pigmentation	

DIAGNOSTIC TESTS

May need to refer for:

- Pap smear
- Other smears and cultures: Gonococcal culture, DNA probe for gonorrhea and chlamydia, wet and dry mounts for other microbes
- Guaiac test of stool

- <u>Urodynamic testing:</u> Comprehensive workup for urinary and/or fecal incontinence
- Sexual dysfunction workup

POSSIBLE NURSING DIAGNOSES

- Pain
- Rape-trauma syndrome
- Self-care deficit, bathing/hygiene
- Sexual dysfunction
- Sexuality patterns, altered

Clinical Alert

- **Signs of sexual assault**
- **Masses**
- **Unusual pain**
- **Postmenopausal bleeding**
- **Infection signs and symptoms**
- **Pregnancy signs**
- **Urinary frequency, urgency, dysuria, or new urinary incontinence**

SAMPLE DOCUMENTATION

Adult

- External genitalia nontender, not inflamed; normal hair distribution. Vaginal mucosa pink, moist, smooth. Cervix nulliparous, pink, without ulcers or nodules, nontender with movement. Pap smear obtained. Uterus palpable, nonenlarged, without masses or tenderness. Ovaries small and nontender. Rectum without hemorrhoids, masses, tenderness. Rectal wall smooth, firm, nontender. Sphincter tone strong.

Child
- Tanner stage I. Labia pink and moist, no discharge.

CLIENT EDUCATION AND HOME HEALTH NOTES

Adult
- Teach good hygiene and prevention of cystitis and vaginitis:
    - Cleanse front to back.
    - Wear loose clothing, as few layers as possible.
    - Wear cotton underpants; avoid pantyhose when possible.
    - Urinate after intercourse.
    - Avoid tub baths, bubble bath, strongly perfumed soaps and powders.
    - Never use vaginal deodorants, deodorized tampons, or pads.
    - Avoid vaginal douches.
    - Drink more fluids (>8 glasses per day) if a history of cystitis.
- Pap smear schedule: After two normal smears, repeat every 2 to 3 years until age 40 if not at high risk (multiple partners, early onset of sexual activity, family history of cancer). Every year after age 40.
- Teach about contraception.
- Teach prevention of STD: Limit activity to one mutually monogamous, uninfected partner; use con-

dom with every exposure; emphasize risk of multiple partners (both STD and cervical cancer).

- Health-care workers at risk for exposure to blood-borne pathogens, who receive blood transfusions, engage in unprotected sexual activity, have multiple sexual partners, or use intravenous drugs should have hepatitis B series. Institutionalized mentally ill persons and those on hemodialysis should also be immunized.

- Teach prevention of HIV:

  - Practice abstinence before marriage. If sexually active, use condoms.

  - Protection necessary for oral sex, rectal intercourse, and vaginal intercourse.

  - Do not have sex with multiple partners or with persons who have had sex with multiple partners, who are intravenous drug users, or who are HIV positive.

  - Do not use drugs. If you do use drugs, do not use IV drugs. If you do use IV drugs, do not share needles.

  - If you have had unprotected sex in the past or used IV drugs, have an HIV test.

Pediatric

- Teach good hygiene as outlined above.

- Teach about contraception and STD prevention as indicated by age and sexual activity.

- Teach parents and child techniques in self-protection; for example, always tell parent or another adult if touched, threatened, or hurt. Assertively refuse to be touched, looked at, or show intimate parts. Tell child that sexual assault is the fault of the adult, not the child.

Geriatric

- Teach about normal changes associated with aging, for example, need for water-soluble lubricant for intercourse.

- Explain that sexual activity is normal into a person's eighties or nineties and beyond if there are no major health problems that interfere.

- Explain that persons with chronic illnesses may need to find alternative positions for sexual intercourse (e.g., side-lying position for client with arthritis) and/or alternative methods for sexual enjoyment (e.g., kissing, caressing, manual stimulation).

- Inform client that fecal and urinary incontinence are treatable conditions and that it is crucial for client to seek help from a health-care provider early. If the health-care provider does not respond to requests for investigation and assistance with incontinence problems, tell client to seek help from a specialist, such as a urologist, a geriatrician, or an advanced practice nurse who specializes in such problems.

- Explain that pelvic examinations by health-care professionals should be performed annually and Pap smears performed as indicated.

- Urinary incontinence (Table 20–1) transient causes:
  - Delirium, acute confusion
  - Urinary tract infection
  - Atrophic vaginitis or urethritis
  - Severe depression
  - Excessive urine production, diuresis
  - Limited mobility
  - Constipation

TABLE 20–1	TYPES OF CHRONIC URINARY INCONTINENCE

- *Stress incontinence:* Involuntary loss of urine with increased abdominal pressure (coughing, sneezing, lifting heavy objects, jumping or running)
- *Urge incontinence:* Involuntary loss of urine associated with an abrupt and strong urge to void (little or no warning, urine loss may be large or small amounts)
- *Overflow incontinence:* Involuntary loss of urine associated with overdistention of the bladder (may present as constant dribbling or frequent small amounts of leakage with stress and urge components)
- *Functional incontinence:* Involuntary loss of urine associated with inability or unwillingness to toilet appropriately because of environmental barriers or physical or cognitive impairments
- *Mixed incontinence:* A combination of different types of incontinence (It is not unusual for a client to experience symptoms of both stress and urge incontinence.)

TABLE 20–2	TREATMENT INTERVENTIONS FOR URINARY INCONTINENCE	
Behavioral	**Medications**	**Surgery**
Bladder training	Anticholinergics	TURP
Bladder retraining	Alpha-adrenergic blockers	Bladder suspension
Environmental manipulation		Repair prolapse
Intermittent catheterization	Antispasmodics	
Pelvic muscle exercises (Kegel exercises)	Cholinergic stimulants	
Biofeedback, electrical stimulation	Topical estrogen	

Source: Adapted from Lueckenotte, A: Pocket Guide to Gerontologic Assessment, ed 3, Mosby, St Louis, 1998.

> • <u>Medications:</u> Sedative hypnotics, diuretics, anti-cholinergics, psychotropics (Table 20–2)

ASSOCIATED COMMUNITY AGENCIES

- <u>Help for Incontinent People:</u> Patient advocacy and education
- <u>National Kidney Foundation:</u> Local screening programs, education, and counseling
- <u>National Kidney and Urologic Diseases Information Clearinghouse:</u> Education

CHAPTER 21

PREGNANCY

HISTORY

Adult
Antepartum

- Age
- Last menstrual period (LMP)
- Menstrual history (See Female Genitourinary System and Rectum, page 298.)
- Contraceptive history (See Female Genitourinary System and Rectum, page 299.)
- Obstetric history: Gravidity, parity, number of preterm births, number of living children. For each previous birth: Gestation, birth weight, length of labor, newborn problems, and problems during pregnancy or labor.
- Number of abortions, spontaneous or induced, and gestation of each
- Health since LMP; if illnesses, nature and treatment

- Accident and/or trauma history since pregnancy or with previous pregnancies. If significant, explore possibility of battering.
- Use of tobacco, alcohol, any drugs since LMP: Note type, amount, frequency.
- Cat in home
- Known genetic or chromosomal abnormalities of either parent or family
- Months attempted conception
- Weight at LMP
- Dietary pattern
- Date of quickening
- Problems with this pregnancy
- Daily routine
- Knowledge of pregnancy and normal changes
- Relationships with father of baby and other family; degree of perceived support
- Assess feelings toward pregnancy, planned or unplanned, current level of acceptance

Intrapartum

- Screening assessment and interview initially performed to determine imminent birth (obstetric triage data)
- Obstetric triage data include:
  - <u>Obstetric history:</u> Gravidity/parity (previous methods of delivery); LMP-estimated date of delivery (EDD) by dates or sonography
  - <u>Primary reason for coming to hospital seeking care:</u> Onset of labor, induction of labor, cesarean section, preterm labor, vaginal bleeding, rupture of membranes

- **Contractions:** Frequency, duration, intensity, onset time, and date
- **Membranes:** Intact, ruptured (date, time, amount, color, odor)
- **Vaginal bleeding:** Mixed with mucus (bloody show), color, amount, onset
- **Cervical exam:** Station, effacement, dilation, presentation
- Fetal heart rate and vital signs
- Admission physical assessment

- **Allergies:** Medications, other (remember Latex sensitivity)
- Additional interview data
  - Recent illness ≤ 14 days before admission
  - Recent exposure to communicable disease
  - **Last oral intake:** Food/solids
  - Medications
  - **Plans for birth and hospital stay:** Support person in labor and delivery; anesthesia: type; adoption; feeding preference; tubal ligation; circumcision
- Psychosocial data
  - Communication deficit
  - Partner/others involved
  - **Basic needs met:** Housing, clothing, food, transportation
  - Free from physical/emotional abuse
  - **Life stress:** Living environment, working, serious illness
  - **Self-care needs:** Able to meet, deficits

- • Emotional status: Happy, ambivalent, anxious, depressed, angry
- Significant prenatal data (the following should be available at admission):
  - Date of first prenatal visit
  - Previous medical history; significant family medical history
  - Prenatal classes/prepared childbirth
  - Lab findings on prenatal record
  - Blood type and Rh; rubella titer; serology; HIV status; hepatitis B surface antigen
  - Maternal problems identified
  - Fetal problems identified

Postpartum

- Delivery date, length of labor, route of delivery, complications, status of infant
- Breast or bottle feeding
- Adequacy or difficulty in self-care (specify)
- Adequacy or difficulty in newborn care: Feeding, bathing, dressing, comforting
- Ability of support person to assist in care of mother and infant
- Contraception planned

Racial and Ethnic

- Perception of pregnancy as natural and healthy or as illness, source of pride or shame
- Meaning and value of children, gender preference
- Roles of mother and father in family
- Common beliefs and practices related to childbearing, for example, raising hands above head

may cause nuchal cord, attending funerals may expose fetus to evil spirits, open windows at night expose fetus to "bad air," pregnant woman attending wedding may bring bad luck to couple, temperature of foods may be significant in postpartum period

- Use of alternative health-care resources such as herbalist, spiritualist, Mexican curandero
- Family and individual roles that may influence decision making, teaching, delivery of care, expression of concerns; for example, mother may defer to father in decision making, father may be reluctant to express fear and anxiety, use of female caregiver may be necessary, significant inclusion of extended family in childbirth

EQUIPMENT

- Stethoscope
- Sphygmomanometer
- Centimeter tape
- Fetoscope (fetal Doppler if available)
- Speculum
- Glove
- Urinalysis for glucose, protein

CLIENT PREPARATION

- Have client in sitting and lying positions.
- Have client empty bladder and obtain clean urine specimen.
- Use supine position as little as possible.

PHYSICAL ASSESSMENT: PREGNANCY

On admission, order of physical assessment is based upon factors surrounding labor, quick assessment of fetal status, fetal position and presentation, and vaginal exam to rule out imminent birth.

Steps	Normal and/or Common Findings	Significant Deviations
ANTEPARTUM ASSESSMENT		
Inspection		
• *Face and head:* Note color, pigmentation, edema.	Chloasma, no edema, nasal stuffiness.	Edema, especially periorbital and around bridge of nose
• *Breasts:* Note size, vascularity, color.	Increased size, visible vessels symmetrical darkened areolar areas.	Pain, redness, warmth
• *Abdomen:* Note size, shape, color striae, umbilical flattening.	Size (Fig. 21–1); ovoid shape, striae, linea nigra may be present; umbilicus flattens after 30 weeks.	Size not appropriate to gestational age
• *Cervix:* Note color, shape of os, discharge.	Dark pink to blue (at 8–12 weeks); softened; os closed in nulliparas; slitlike opening in multiparas; no bleeding; increased white creamy discharge.	Frank bleeding not associated with examination or intercourse
• Musculoskeletal.	Increased lumbar curve and waddling gait in last trimester; mild dependent edema with prolonged standing.	Marked dependent edema
Palpation		
• *Abdomen:* Note size, pain.	Fundal height palpable after 12–13 weeks (see Fig. 21–1).	Fundal height not appropriate to gestational age; painful to palpate

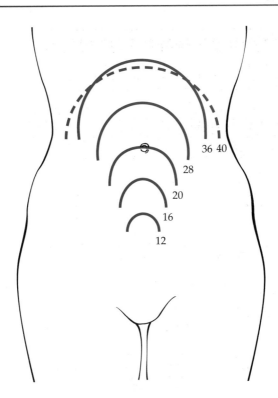

FIGURE 21–1

Fundal heights and gestation.

PHYSICAL ASSESSMENT: PREGNANCY

(Continued)

Steps	Normal and/or Common Findings	Significant Deviations
ANTEPARTUM ASSESSMENT		
• *Neurologic:* Note reflex irritability.	Reflexes +2. No clonus.	Reflexes +3 or +4; clonus of ankle
Auscultation		
• *Heart:* Note rate, other sounds.	Rate may increase 10–15 beats per minute. May have short systolic murmurs.	Tachycardia; marked murmurs, palpitations
• *Blood pressure.*	First and third trimesters at prepregnant level; falls in second trimester.	>140/90 or systolic increase of 30 mm Hg; diastolic increase of 15 mm Hg (If elevated, turn to left side; test urine for protein.)
• *Fetal heart:* Note rate, rhythm, location (on mother's abdomen as RUQ, RLQ, LUQ, LLQ).	>160 at 12 weeks decreasing to 110–160 in late pregnancy; increases 15 beats per minute with activity; regular or slightly irregular rhythm.	Not audible after 12 weeks with Doppler; not audible after 18–20 weeks with fetoscope Rate <110–120 in last trimester; no increase in rate with fetal movement; pattern or irregularity
INITIAL INTRAPARTUM ASSESSMENT		
Inspection		
• *General appearance:* Look for signs of distress.	Appearance and behavior varies depending on stage and phase of labor	Birth practices in different cultures; vary with ethnic groups and different religions

PHYSICAL ASSESSMENT: PREGNANCY

(Continued)

Steps	Normal and/or Common Findings	Significant Deviations
INITIAL INTRAPARTUM ASSESSMENT		
• *Face and head:* Note color, edema.	No edema, nasal stuffiness.	*Edema:* especially periorbital and around bridge of nose
• *Breasts:* Note size, vascularity, color.	Increased size, visible vessels symmetrical, darkened, areolar areas.	*Pain, redness, warmth*
• *Abdomen:* Note size, shape, color, striae, umbilicus flattening.	*Size:* ovoid shape, striae, linea nigra may be present; umbilicus flattens after 30 weeks.	*Size not appropriate to gestational age*
Palpation • *Abdomen:* Note size, fetal positioning/presentation, pain, uterine activity.	Fundal height palpation initially done for size estimation, Leopold's maneuvers. Evaluation of labor contractions.	Fundal height not appropriate to gestational age; fetal presentation other than vertex; uterine tone rigid without relaxing; extremely painful to palpate
• *Neurologic:* Note reflex irritability.	Reflexes +2; no clonus.	*Reflexes +3 or +4; clonus of ankle*
• *Vaginal examination:* Cervical dilation and effacement; fetal station and presentation. Inspection of vaginal secretions.	Vaginal examination dependent on stage and phase of labor.	Bloody show in absence of pain; abnormal fetal presentation; presence of umbilical cord with presenting part; amniotic fluid with foul odor or meconium stained

Table continued on following page

PHYSICAL ASSESSMENT: PREGNANCY

(Continued)

Steps	Normal and/or Common Findings	Significant Deviations
INITIAL INTRAPARTUM ASSESSMENT		
Auscultation		
• *Heart:* Note rate, rhythm, presence of murmur.	Rate may increase 10–15 beats per minute above non-pregnant rate. May have short systolic murmur.	Tachycardia; marked murmurs
• *Blood pressure:* See vital signs.	Will increase during contractions—check without contraction for accuracy.	Palpitations Blood pressure readings of ≥30 mm Hg systolic baseline, ≥15 mm Hg diastolic baseline or reading of 140/90 mm Hg × 2–6 hours apart
• *Lungs:* Note breath sounds, adventitious sounds.	Lung fields clear.	Any adventitious breath sounds; hyperventilation
• *Fetal heart (FHR):* Note rate, rhythm, location (on mother's abdomen as RUQ, RLQ, LUQ, LLQ), FHR response to contractions.	*Reassuring FHR patterns:* Baseline 120–160 beats per minute (110 if >40 weeks); average variability 6–10 beats per minute; no nonreassuring periodic changes. Acceleration of FHR with fetal movement reassuring.	Rate <110–120 beats per minute; variability consistently <6 beats per minute; no increase in rate with fetal activity. *Nonreassuring periodic changes:* FHR decelerations that begin after peak of contraction, lasting after contraction is over.

PHYSICAL ASSESSMENT: PREGNANCY

(Continued)

Steps	Normal and/or Common Findings	Significant Deviations
INITIAL INTRAPARTUM ASSESSMENT		
		Severe variable decelerations, FHR <60 beats per minute ≥60 seconds or variable decelerations with increasing baseline and decreasing variability associated with neonatal depression.
Vital signs • Initial assessment should be used as baseline, as labor progresses.	Temperature monitored every 4 hours; if membranes ruptured, every 2 hours. Pulse and respiration monitored every 30–60 minutes in latent phase (early labor); every 15–30 minutes in transition phase. Blood pressure (should be at prepregnant level by 28 weeks) monitored same as pulse and respiration (if epidural anesthetic, every 15 minutes).	Temperature >100. Possible infection or fluid deficit Tachycardia, tachypnea >140/90 or systolic increase of 30 mm Hg; diastolic increase of 15 mm Hg (if elevated, turn to left side, test urine for protein).

Table continued on following page

PHYSICAL ASSESSMENT: PREGNANCY *(Continued)*

INTRAPARTUM: EXPECTED MATERNAL PROGRESS DURING LABOR

	Stage 1*†			Stage 2‡	Stage 3	Stage 4
• Dilatation	0–3 cm (latent)	4–7 cm (active)	8–10 cm (transition)	Pushing—delivery of baby	Placental expulsion	2 hours postpartum
• Duration	About 6–8 hours	About 3–6 hours	About 20–40 minutes	Nullipara 25–75 minutes; average 57 minutes / Multipara 13–17 minutes; average 14	5–30 minutes	
• Contractions Strength	Mild to moderate	Moderate to strong	Strong to very strong	Strong to very strong	Very strong	Afterbirth pains / Mild
Rhythm Frequency	Irregular 5–30 minutes apart	More regular 3–5 minutes apart	Regular 2–3 minutes apart	Regular 2–3 minutes apart	Regular 1½–3 minutes apart	Irregular / Uterus must remain firm to decrease postpartum bleeding
Duration	30–45 seconds	40–70 seconds	45–90 seconds	90 seconds	60–90 seconds	
• Descent station of presenting past show	Nullip: 0 / Multip: 0–2 cm	Varies +1 cm to +2 cm	Varies +2 cm to +3 cm	0 to +2 → +4 at birth		

Color	Brown discharge, mucus plug or pale pink mucus	Pink to bloody mucus	Bloody mucus	Significant increase in dark red bloody show → Fetal head at introitus; bloody show at birth	Gushing of dark blood; cord lengthens	Lochia-rubra-like heavy menses with clots
Amount	Scant	Scant to moderate	Copious			
• Behavior and appearance	Excited—Self-control, thinking of baby, fairly well controlled; follows directions	More serious, more apprehensive; wants encouragement; focused inwardly; some difficulty following directions	Pain—Severe, frustration, fear of loss of control; irritable; nausea and vomiting; feels need to defecate	Relief, fatigue—Sleepy; "worst is over"; feels in control → extreme pain; decreased ability to listen; focused on giving birth, extreme excitement after delivery of head	Relief—Crying, laughing, concern for baby	Many factors affect mother: low energy level, physical comfort, health of newborn; transitioning

*In nullipara women, effacement usually complete before dilatation begins; in multipara women effacement and dilatation occur simultaneously.

Average total duration of stage 1 nullipara 10–16 hours; multipara 6–10 hours.

†Duration of first and second stage of labor influenced by parity, maternal position and activity. Nullipara's labor > multipara's labor.

‡Length of time during second stage lengthens with epidural anesthesia.

Table continued on following page

PHYSICAL ASSESSMENT: PREGNANCY

(Continued)

Steps	Normal and/or Common Findings	Significant Deviations
POSTPARTUM ASSESSMENT		
Inspection		
• *Breasts:* Note color, feeding ability.	No redness; infant able to root, grasp areolar tissue in mouth, suck 5 minutes each side first days in at least two positions	Redness Infant unable to suck 5 minutes each side
• *Abdomen:* Note uterine, bladder positions.	Not visible or midline, below umbilicus	Easily visible above umbilicus or deviated laterally
• *Perineum:* Note color, integrity, swelling, drainage.	Slight redness, mild edema, lochia appropriate to time (rubra to serosa)	Bright red or unilateral redness; continued lochia rubra beyond first days; strong odor
	If episiotomy, no signs of infection of incision If hemorrhoids, may be swollen	Bright red bleeding; signs of infection of episiotomy
Palpation		
• *Breast* (wash hands before touching): Note warmth, hard areas, tenderness or pain.	Mild uniform warmth; no masses; some tenderness, especially nipples	Hot areas, hardened areas, painful to touch
• *Abdomen:* Note fundal height, firmness; bladder, tenderness.	*Day 1:* At umbilicus, firm *Day 2:* Umbilicus +1–2 cm *Day 3:* At umbilicus *Day 4:* Steady decrease Bladder not palpable	Fundus boggy, elevated, deviated laterally; bladder palpable with suprapubic tenderness

PHYSICAL ASSESSMENT: PREGNANCY

(Continued)

Steps	Normal and/or Common Findings	Significant Deviations
POSTPARTUM ASSESSMENT		
• *Legs:* Gently palpate calves for heat, tenderness. Dorsiflex ankle, and ask client if pain felt in calf.	No heat No pain (negative Homans' sign)	Heat, pain on dorsiflexion (positive Homans' sign)
• *Skin:* Note temperature, moisture.	Warm (oral temperature <100.4°F); increased perspiration	Temperature >100.4°F

DIAGNOSTIC TESTS

May need to refer for:

- Initial prenatal tests include: CBC, urinalysis, serology, HIV, rubella screen, blood type, Rh and antibody screen, hepatitis B surface antigen, DNA probe for chlamydia and gonorrhea, Pap smear. Possibly culture for group B beta streptococcus.
- Diabetic screen in 2nd trimester
- Ultrasonography
- Pelvimetry

POSSIBLE NURSING DIAGNOSES

- Sleep pattern disturbance
- Breastfeeding, effective, ineffective
- Knowledge deficit (learning need) (specify)

- Fatigue
- Growth and development, altered
- Body image disturbance
- Nutrition: altered, more or less than body requirements
- Family processes, altered

Clinical Alert

- Elevated blood pressure, facial edema, proteinuria, glucosuria, headache
- Fetal heart rate abnormalities
- Uterine growth disproportionate to gestational age
- Mother's report of decreased fetal movement
- Bleeding not associated with examination or intercourse
- Abdominal pain

SAMPLE DOCUMENTATION

Age 33; G-2, P-1, LC-1, Ab-0. Approximately 22 weeks gestation (LMP 5/26; EDD 2/28). Fundus at umbilicus 20 cm, FHT 170 LLQ. Urine neg/neg; weight 158; BP 100/70. Bimanual: Cervix closed, soft, thick. Speculum: Cervix closed, without lesions or drainage.

CLIENT AND FAMILY EDUCATION AND HOME HEALTH NOTES

- Teach normal changes of pregnancy, and maternal and fetal development.

- Review dietary needs every month. Assess with recall if weight gain too much or too little.

- Encourage moderate exercise (e.g., walking, swimming) and rest.

- Explain that normal weight gain is from 24 to 32 pounds. During first 28 weeks, client should gain ½ to ¾ pound per week; then she should gain from 1 to 1½ pounds per week.

- Teach danger signs in pregnancy.

- Teach warning signs of labor.

- Teach infant care and infant normal growth and development.

- Discuss breast-feeding and provide information and support. Provide information about bottle feeding if desired.

- Discuss return to sexual activity.

- Teach client when to see health-care provider postpartum (baby is normally seen at 2 weeks, mother at 6 weeks).

- Assess and provide information about sibling preparation.

- Assess adequacy of infant care supplies:
  - Crib or bassinet
  - Car seat
  - Infant clothing, diapers, feeding materials

- Assess availability of support person for labor and postpartum.

ASSOCIATED COMMUNITY AGENCIES

Assess the need for and refer as appropriate to:

- Prenatal parenting classes

- Family resource centers
- Licensed breastfeeding specialists
- Local support agencies for new parents and breast-feeding mothers
- Supplemental Nutrition Program for Women, Infants, and Children (WIC)
- Food stamps
- Temporary Aid to Needy Families (TANF)
- LaLeche League
- Parenting classes

NANDA-Approved Nursing Diagnoses

This list represents the NANDA-approved nursing diagnoses for clinical use and testing (1999–2000).

- ACTIVITY/REST
  Activity intolerance
  Activity intolerance, risk for
  Disuse syndrome, risk for
  Diversional activity deficit
  Fatigue
  Mobility, impaired bed
  Mobility, impaired wheelchair
  Sleep deprivation
  Sleep pattern disturbance
  Transfer ability, impaired
  Walking, impaired

- CIRCULATION
  Adaptive capacity; intracranial, decreased
  [Autonomic] dysreflexia
  Autonomic dysreflexia, risk for
  Cardiac output, decreased
  Tissue perfusion, altered

- EGO INTEGRITY
  Adjustment, impaired
  Anxiety (specify level)
  Anxiety, death
  Body image disturbance
  Coping, defensive
  Coping, individual, ineffective
  Decisional conflict (specify)

Source: **Taber's Cyclopedic Medical Dictionary, ed 19. FA Davis, Philadelphia, 2001, with permission. An asterisk denotes a newly approved diagnosis.**

Denial, ineffective
Energy field disturbance
Fear
Grieving, anticipatory
Grieving, dysfunctional
Hopelessness
Personal identity disturbance
Post-trauma syndrome
Post-trauma syndrome, risk for
Powerlessness
*Powerlessness, risk for
Rape-trauma syndrome
Rape-trauma syndrome: compound reaction
Rape-trauma syndrome: silent reaction
Relocation stress syndrome
*Relocation stress syndrome, risk for
Self-esteem, chronic low
Self-esteem disturbance
*Self-esteem, risk for situational low
Self-esteem, situational low
Sorrow, chronic
Spiritual distress (distress of the human spirit)
Spiritual distress, risk for
Spiritual well-being, potential for enhanced

- ELIMINATION
Bowel incontinence
Constipation
Constipation, perceived
*Constipation, risk for
Diarrhea
Urinary elimination, altered
Urinary incontinence, functional
Urinary incontinence, reflex
Urinary incontinence, risk for urge
[Urinary] incontinence, stress
[Urinary] incontinence, total
[Urinary] incontinence, urge
Urinary retention

- FOOD/FLUID
Breastfeeding, effective
Breastfeeding, ineffective
Breastfeeding, interrupted
Dentition, altered

Failure to thrive, adult
Fluid volume deficit
Fluid volume excess
Fluid volume, risk for deficit
Fluid volume, risk for imbalance
Infant feeding pattern, ineffective
Nausea
Nutrition: altered, less than body requirements
Nutrition: altered, more than body requirements
Nutrition: altered, risk for more than body requirements
Oral mucous membrane, altered
Swallowing, impaired

- HYGIENE
  Self-care deficit (specify)

- NEUROSENSORY
  Confusion, acute
  Confusion, chronic
  Infant behavior, disorganized
  Infant behavior, organized, potential for enhancement
  Infant behavior, risk for disorganized
  Memory, impaired
  Peripheral neurovascular, risk for dysfunction
  Sensory/perceptual alterations (specify)
  Thought processes, altered
  Unilateral neglect

- PAIN/DISCOMFORT
  Pain
  Pain, chronic

- RESPIRATION
  Airway clearance, ineffective
  Aspiration, risk for
  Breathing pattern, ineffective
  Gas exchange, impaired
  Spontaneous ventilation: inability to sustain
  Ventilatory weaning response, dysfunctional

- SAFETY
  Body temperature, altered, risk for
  Environmental interpretation syndrome, impaired
  *Falls, risk for
  Health maintenance, altered
  Home maintenance management, impaired

Hyperthermia
Hypothermia
Infection, risk for
Injury, risk for
Latex allergy response
Latex allergy response, risk for
Mobility, impaired physical
Perioperative positioning injury, risk for
Poisoning, risk for
Protection, altered
*Self-mutilation
Self-mutilation, risk for
Skin integrity, impaired
Skin integrity, risk for impaired
Suffocation, risk for
*Suicide, risk for
Surgical recovery, delayed
Thermoregulation, ineffective
Tissue integrity, impaired
Trauma, risk for
Violence, [actual] risk for directed at others
Violence, [actual] risk for self-directed
*Wandering (specify sporadic or continual)

- SEXUALITY (COMPONENT OF EGO INTEGRITY AND SOCIAL INTERACTION)
  Sexual dysfunction
  Sexuality patterns, altered

- SOCIAL INTERACTION
  Caregiver role strain
  Caregiver role strain, risk for
  Communication, impaired verbal
  Community coping, ineffective
  Community coping, potential for enhanced
  Family coping, ineffective, compromised
  Family coping, ineffective, disabling
  Family coping, potential for growth
  Family processes, altered
  Family processes, altered: alcoholism
  Loneliness, risk for
  *Parent/infant attachment, risk for insecure
  Parent/infant/child attachment, risk for, altered
  Parental role conflict
  Parenting, altered
  Parenting, risk for, altered

Role performance, altered
Social interaction, impaired
Social isolation

- TEACHING/LEARNING
Development, risk for, altered
Growth and development, altered
Growth, risk for, altered
Health-seeking behaviors (specify)
Knowledge deficit (specify)
Noncompliance (specify)
Therapeutic regimen: community, ineffective management
Therapeutic regimen: families, ineffective management
Therapeutic regimen: individual, effective management
Therapeutic regimen: (individuals), ineffective management

Age Categories and Labels and Words Used for Older People

Age Categories

Young-old	65–74
Middle-old	75–84
Old-old	85–94
Elite-old	95 and older

Functional status is more important than chronological age.

Categories provided by the National Institute on Aging, August 30, 1994.

Many words and terms should not be used when talking with, when talking about, or when writing about disabled or older people. Many of the terms are *disrespectful* and *demeaning*. Other terms have *unclear meanings* open to various interpretations:

DO NOT USE	SUBSTITUTE
• Adult day care (similar to child care)	Adult day services (may include needed health care)
• Adult diaper (implies being a baby)	Pants, pads, briefs, trade name (product)
• Afflicted	Affected by
• Aged	Older people

Source: Adapted from Hogstel, MO: Community Resources for Older Adults: A Guide for Case Managers. St Louis: Mosby, 1998, with permission.

DO NOT USE	SUBSTITUTE
• Bed-bound (not tied to the bed)	In bed much of the time
• Bed sore	Pressure ulcer (area)
• Bib	Clothes protector
• Cerebral-palsied	People with cerebral palsy
• Childish, childlike	None (never use)
• Convalescent home	Nursing facility (home)
• Crazy	Mentally ill (often with a physical cause)
• Crippled	Disabled
• Deaf and dumb	Hearing and speech impaired
• Elderly (implies 50–110 all alike)	Older people
• First name or familial title (Granny)	Only if family, friend, or by request
• Formula (relates to babies)	Nutritional supplement
• Frail, fragile (what does this mean?)	Disabled (or describe specific problem)
• Golden agers	None (never use)
• Greedy geezers (odd character)	None (never use)
• Handicapped	Disabled
• Homebound, shut-in (not tied to the house)	Rarely leaves home
• Honey, dearie, sweetie, Grandpa, Grandma	Mr., Ms.
• Incompetent	Incapacitated (legal term)
• Little old lady/man	Older woman/man
• Older generation	Older people
• Oldsters	Older people
• Old timer's disease (implying Alzheimer's)	None (never use)
• Poor	Low income
• Rest home	Nursing facility (home)
• Role reversal (dependent parent becomes child)	Role reversal does not occur (a mature adult-to-adult relationship)
• Senile	None (never use)
• Senior	Older adult
• Senior moment (implies forgetfulness)	Never use (all ages forget at times)
• Sitter (used for babies)	Companion
• Suffers (from a disease)	Has a disease

DO NOT USE	SUBSTITUTE
• Symptoms/problems due to age	Diagnose and treat
• Victim (of a disease)	None (never use)
• Wheelchair-bound (not tied to the wheelchair)	Wheelchair user
• Young man/lady—when obviously older	None (never use)

NOTE: Some words have been contributed by REACH, a Resource Center on Independent Living in Forth Worth, TX.

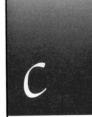

Sample Health History Form

Date _____ Name _____

Room _____ Sex: M F

Address _____

Telephone number _____

Private home _____ Apartment _____

Retirement center _____ Nursing facility _____

Date of birth _____ Age _____

Date of admission _____ Date of surgery _____

Marital status: M W S D

If widowed, how long? _____

Retired _____ Occupation _____

Social Security number _____

Medicare number _____

Medicaid number _____

Source: Adapted from Nursing History Form 584, Harris School of
    Nursing, Texas Christian University, Fort Worth, TX, 2000,
    with permission.

Insurance name _____

Number ___._____

Religious preference _____

Contact in emergency _____

Reason for seeking care (chief complaint) _____

_____

History of present illness/condition/surgery

_____

_____

_____

Patient's understanding of current condition _____

_____

Current diet _____

Medications currently prescribed _____

_____

Past health/medical history

_____

_____

_____

Allergies (food, medicines, environmental) _____

_____

Medications and treatments at home _____

_____

Chemical use

Number of cigarettes per day _____

Other tobacco per day _____

Number of years smoked _____

Amount of coffee/tea/carbonated beverages per day _____

Amount of alcoholic drinks per day _____

Type _____

Use of other substances _____

_____

Rest and sleep patterns

Hours worked per day _____ Rest periods or naps (when,

Hours of sleep per night _____

Medications used to aid sleep _____

Other measures to aid sleep _____

Sleep problems _____

_____

Mobility and exercise patterns

Type of activity/exercise _____

Amount (times per week, minutes per day) _____

Restrictions/mechanical aids/prostheses/wheelchair/walker/ bedrails

_____

Ability to care for self _____

_____

Diet

                         Breakfast   Lunch   Dinner   Snacks

24-hour recall of
  previous day

Usual time of
  meals at home

Ability to feed self _____ Dentures _____

Dietary restrictions/dislikes, difficulty _____

Fluid intake per day (type and amount) _____

Elimination routines, frequency, problems, aids

Bowel _____

_____

Urinary _____

_____

Communication

Ability to understand English _____

Language spoken _____

Hearing _____ Sight _____ Aids _____

Educational level _____

Ability to speak _____

Orientation: Person _____   Time _____

Place _____

Present emotional state _____

Activities

Hobbies _____

Part-time employment _____

Volunteer work _____

Other _____

Family history
Composition
  Number in household
  Roles
Primary support system
History of family health/illness
Other pertinent data

Environmental history

REVIEW OF SYSTEMS

System	History	Not Asked
General overview		
Skin/hair/nails		

REVIEW OF SYSTEMS *(Continued)*

System	History	Not Asked
Head and Neck		
Eyes		
Ears		
Nose/sinus		
Mouth/throat		
Respiratory		
Cardiovascular		

REVIEW OF SYSTEMS *(Continued)*

System	History	Not Asked
Gastrointestinal		
Breasts/axillae		
Genitourinary		
Musculoskeletal		
Neurologic		
Other pertinent data		

Sample Mental Status Flow Sheet

KEY

✓ Intact

L Limited

D Difficult

◊ Absent

SUGGESTED SCHEDULE

Each shift or daily (hospital)
Weekly (nursing facility)
Monthly (nursing facility, home health agency)

Assessment*	Each Shift or Daily			or	Weekly						or	Monthly				
	Date	Date	Date		Date		Date		Date			Date		Date		
	Time	Time	Time		A.M.	P.M.	A.M.	P.M.	A.M.	P.M.		A.M.	P.M.	A.M.	P.M.	
1. Oriented to person																
a. First name																
b. Last name																
2. Oriented to place																
a. City																
b. State																
c. Name of facility																
d. Address of facility																
3. Oriented to time																
a. Year																
b. Month																
c. Date of month																
d. Day of week																
e. A.M. or P.M.																

Assessment*	Each Shift or Daily						or	Weekly				or	Monthly			
	Date	Date	Date					Date		Date			Date		Date	
	Time	Time	Time					A.M.	P.M.	A.M.	P.M.		A.M.	P.M.	A.M.	P.M.
4. Memory a. Immediate (minutes): Name three objects and ask to repeat in several minutes.																
b. Recent (days): Ask what the person did yesterday afternoon.																
c. Remote (years): Ask about year of marriage or president during World War II.																
d. Old (not recalled recently): Ask names of teachers from grade school.																

Table continued on following page

353

Assessment*	Each Shift or Daily						or	Weekly						or	Monthly			
	Date		Date		Date			Date		Date		Date			Date		Date	
	Time		Time		Time			A.M.	P.M.	A.M.	P.M.	A.M.	P.M.		A.M.	P.M.	A.M.	P.M.
5. Intelligence a. Vocabulary: Ask to name several objects such as a pencil.																		
b. Calculations: Ask to add or subtract two numbers.																		
c. Construction: Ask to draw the face of a clock.																		

354

Assessment*	Each Shift or Daily			or				Weekly								or				Monthly							
	Date	Date	Date		Date		Date		Date		Date		Date				Date		Date		Date	
	Time	Time	Time		A.M.	P.M.	A.M.	P.M.	A.M.	P.M.	A.M.	P.M.	A.M.	P.M.	A.M.	P.M.		A.M.	P.M.	A.M.	P.M.	A.M.	P.M.
6. Abstract thinking a. Proverbs: Ask the meaning of a proverb such as "When it rains, it pours."																							
b. Analogies: Ask how an apple and an orange are alike.																							
7. Mental status test score a. SPMSQ† b. Other																							

*Suggestions for assessment are only examples. Many other similar ones may be used.
†See Appendix E.
Source: Adapted from Hogstel, MO: Assessing mental status. J Geront Nurs 17(5):43, 1991, with permission.

355

The Folstein Mini-Mental State Examination (test of cognitive function)

Maximum Score	Score	Orientation
5	( )	What is the (year)(season)(date)(day)(month)?
5	( )	Where are we: (state)(county)(town)(hospital)(floor)?
		Registration
3	( )	Name 3 objects: 1 second to say each. Then ask the patient all 3 after you have said them. Give 1 point for each correct answer. Then repeat them until he learns all 3. Count trials and record. Trials _____
		Attention and Calculation
5	( )	Serial 7's. 1 point for each correct. Stop after 5 answers. Alternatively spell "world" backwards.

		Recall
3	( )	Ask for 3 objects repeated above. Give 1 point for each correct.
		Language
2	( )	Name a pencil and watch.
1	( )	Repeat the following: "No ifs, ands, or buts."
3	( )	Follow a 3 stage command: "Take a paper in your right hand, fold it in half, and put it on the floor."
1	( )	Read and obey the following:
		CLOSE YOUR EYES
1	( )	Write a sentence.
1	( )	Copy design.
30		

ASSESS level of consciousness along a
continuum _____
            alert drowsy stupor coma

Source: Adapted from Folstein, MF, Folstein, SE, and McHugh,
PR: Mini-mental state. Journal of Psychiatric Research,
12(1):196–197, 1975. Used with permission.

INSTRUCTIONS FOR ADMINISTRATION OF MINI-MENTAL STATE EXAMINATION

Orientation

Ask for the date. Then ask specifically for parts omitted, e.g., "Can you also tell me what season it is?" One point for each correct.

Ask in turn "Can you tell me the name of this hospital?" (town, county, etc.). One point for each correct.

Registration

Ask the patient if you may test his memory. Then say the names of three unrelated objects, clearly and slowly, about one second for each. After you have said all three, ask him to repeat them. This first repetition determines his score (0–3) but keep saying them until he can repeat all three, up to six trials. If he does not eventually learn all three, recall cannot be meaningfully tested.

Attention and Calculation

Ask the patient to begin with 100 and count backwards by 7. Stop after 5 subtractions (93, 86, 79, 72, 65). Score the total number of correct answers.

If the patient cannot or will not perform this task, ask him to spell the word "world" backwards. The score is the number of letters in correct order, e.g., dlrow = 5, dlorw = 3.

Recall

Ask the patient if he can recall the three words you previously asked him to remember. Score 0–3.

Language

Naming: Show the patient a wrist watch and ask him what it is. Repeat for pencil. Score 0–2.

Repetition: Ask the patient to repeat the sentence after you. Allow only one trial. Score 0 or 1.

3-Stage command: Give the patient a piece of plain blank paper and repeat the command. Score 1 point for each part correctly executed (Folstein, et al., 1975, p. 197).

Scoring: A score of 20 or less has been found "only in patients with dementia, delirium, schizophrenia or affective disorders" (Folstein, et al., 1975, p. 196). The MMS is not timed and should only take about 5–10 minutes (Folstein, et al., 1975, p. 189).

NOTE: Some changes in administration and scoring have occurred over the years based on research. Gallo, Reichel, and Andersen (1995, p. 33) used a "cutoff score of 24 . . . to indicate dementia." Scores may vary based on formal education completed and age.

REFERENCES

Folstein, MF, Folstein, SE, and McHugh, PR: Mini-mental state. Journal of Psychiatric Research, 12(1):189–198, 1975.
Gallo, JJ, Reichel, W, and Andersen, LM: Handbook of Geriatric Assessment. Aspen, Gaithersburg, MD, 1995.

Katz Index of Independence in Activities of Daily Living

The Index of Independence in Activities of Daily Living (ADLs) is based on an evaluation of the functional independence or dependence of patients in bathing, dressing, going to toilet, transferring, continence, and feeding. Specific definitions of functional independence and dependence appear after the index.

EVALUATION FORM

Name _____ Date of evaluation _____

For each area of functioning listed below, check the one description that best applies. (The word *assistance* means supervision, direction of personal assistance.)

Bathing—either sponge bath, tub bath, or shower.

☐ Receives no assistance (gets into and out of tub by self if tub is usual means of bathing)

☐ Receives assistance in bathing only one part of the body (such as back or a leg)

☐ Receives assistance in bathing more than one part of the body (or not bathed)

Source: Adapted from Katz, S, Ford, AB, Moskowitz, RW, et al: Studies of illness in the aged: The Index of ADL. JAMA 185:914–919, 1963, with permission.

Dressing—gets clothes from closets and drawers including under-clothes and outer garments and uses fasteners (including braces if worn).

☐ Gets clothes and gets completely dressed without assistance

☐ Gets clothes and gets dressed without assistance except for assistance in tying shoes

☐ Receives assistance in getting clothes or in getting dressed, or stays partly or completely undressed

Toileting—going to the "toilet room" for bowel and urine elimination; cleaning self after elimination, and arranging clothes.

☐ Goes to the "toilet room," cleans self, and arranges clothes without assistance (may use for support such object as cane, walker, or wheelchair and may manage night bedpan or commode, emptying same in morning)

☐ Receives assistance in going to "toilet room" or in cleansing self or in arranging clothes after elimination or in use of night bedpan or commode

☐ Does not go to room termed "toilet" for the elimination process

Transfers*

☐ Moves into and out of bed as well as into and out of chair without assistance (may be using object for support such as cane or walker)

☐ Moves into or out of bed or chair with assistance

☐ Does not get out of bed

*Ask the client to show you the bathroom and medications in another room to assess ability to transfer, walk, and communicate.

Continence

☐ Controls urination and bowel movement completely by self

☐ Has occasional "accidents"

☐ Supervision to keep urine or bowel control; catheter used or is incontinent

Feeding

☐ Feeds self without assistance

☐ Feeds self except for getting assistance in cutting meat or buttering bread

☐ Receives assistance in feeding or is fed partly or completely by using tubes or intravenous fluids

Convert the above data into an overall ADL grade based on the following definitions. Note that the intermediate description may be dependent for some functions and independent for others.

A   Independent in feeding, continence, transferring, going to toilet, dressing, and bathing

B   Independent in all but one of these functions

C   Independent in all but bathing and one additional function

D   Independent in all but bathing, dressing, and one additional function

F   Independent in all but bathing, dressing, going to toilet, transferring, and one additional function

G   Dependent in all six functions

Other   Dependent in at least two functions but not classifiable as C, D, E, or F

Definitions

Independence means without supervision, direction, or active personal assistance, except as specifically noted below. This is based on actual status and not on ability. A client who refuses to perform a function is considered as not performing the function, even though he or she is deemed able.

Bathing (Sponge, Shower, or Tub)

Independent. Assistance only in bathing a single part (as back or disabled extremity) or bathes self completely

Dependent. Assistance in bathing more than one part of body; assistance in getting into or out of tub or does not bathe self

Dressing

Independent. Gets clothes from closets and drawers; puts on clothes, outer garments, braces; manages fasteners (Act of tying shoes is excluded.)

Dependent. Does not dress self or remains partly undressed

Going to Toilet

Independent. Gets to toilet; gets on and off toilet; arranges clothes; cleans organs of excretion; may manage own bedpan used at night only and may or may not be using mechanical supports

Dependent. Uses bedpan or commode or receives assistance in getting to and using toilet

Transfer

Independent. Moves into and out of bed independently and moves into and out of chair independently; may or may not be using mechanical supports

Dependent. Assistance in moving into or out of bed and/or chair; does not perform one or more transfers

Continence

Independent. Urination and defecation entirely self-controlled

Dependent. Partial or total incontinence in urination or defecation; partial or total control by enemas, catheters, or regulated use of urinals and/or bedpans

Feeding

Independent. Gets food from plate or its equivalent into mouth (Precutting of meat and preparation of food, such as buttering bread, are excluded from evaluation.)

Dependent. Assistance in act of feeding (see above); does not eat at all or receives parenteral feeding

Apgar Scoring System: A Rapid Assessment Technique to Determine Need for Resuscitation at 1 and 5 Minutes after Birth

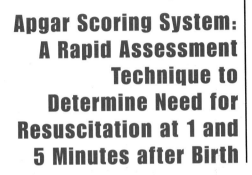

	0	1	2
Heart rate	None	<100	>100
Respiration	None	Slow or irregular	Cries or makes good effort
Muscle tone	Flaccid	Mild flexion of extremities	Active movement
Reflex response (insert catheter in nostril after clearing oropharynx)	No response	Slow movement or grimaces	Cries, coughs, or sneezes
Color*	Blue, pale	Extremities blue, body pink	Completely pink

*Skin color or its absence may not be a reliable guide in nonwhites, although melanin is less apparent at birth than later.

Table continued on following page

Source: Adapted from Taber's Cyclopedic Medical Dictionary, ed 18. FA Davis, Philadelphia, 1997, pp 131–132, with permission.

Scoring: Score each assessment area as 0, 1, or 2, based on the above criteria. Add the total score including all areas.

Interpretation:

    0–3 = poor condition

    4–6 = fair condition

    7–10 = good to excellent condition

Immunization Schedule: Pediatric and Adult

VACCINES

Name	Age Administered	Booster Schedule	Comments
CG (bacillus of Calmette and Guérin)	In epidemic conditions, administered to infants as soon as possible after birth.	None.	The only contraindications are symptomatic human immunodeficiency virus (HIV) infection or other illnesses known to suppress immunity.
Cholera	See Comments.	Every 3 to 6 months for those who remain in epidemic areas.	Only those traveling to countries where cholera is present need to be vaccinated. Whole cell vaccines provide partial protection for 3 to 6 months.

Table continued on following page

Name	Age Administered	Booster Schedule	Comments
DPT (diphtheria, pertussis, tetanus)	At 2, 4, 6, and 15–18 months. A fifth dose may be given at 4–6 years.	Tetanus and diphtheria immunization every 10 years, esp. for people over 50. Persons who have received five doses of tetanus toxoid in childhood may not need a booster until age 50.	Tetanus booster may be required following a wound even though all routine and booster immunizations have been received. Booster of diphtheria toxoid should be given if child under 6 is exposed to diphtheria. Vaccine is contraindicated in cases of acute infection, previous central nervous system damage, or convulsions.
Haemophilus influenzae b (polysaccharide or conjugate)	At 2 months, 4 months, discretionally at 6 months, and at 12–15 months.	None.	Important: Check package insert for appropriate scheduling information. Booster doses may be required.
Hepatitis B	At birth, 2 months, and 6–18 months, or at 1–2 months, 4 months, and 6–18 months.	None.	Recommended as a routine childhood vaccine. All health-care workers should receive it. Immune

Table continued on following page

Name	Age Administered	Booster Schedule	Comments
	All ages if risk is present.		globulin or hepatitis B globulin may be given to produce passive immunity in exposed contacts. They are contraindicated for those allergic to yeast products.
Influenza (flu)	All ages.	Annually, given prior to time influenza is expected.	Recommended for older adults, healthcare professionals, residents of long-term care facilities, and those of any age who have chronic disease of the heart or lungs, metabolic diseases such as diabetes, or immunosuppression.
MMR (measles [live attenuated rubeola], mumps, rubella)	12–15 months.	4–6 years or 11–12 years.	Vaccine will usually prevent measles if given within 2 days after a child has been exposed to the disease. Not given to adults. Con-

Table continued on following page

Name	Age Administered	Booster Schedule	Comments
			traindicated for those with allergy to egg or neomycin, active infection, or severe immunosuppression.
Plague	See Comments.	See Comments.	Recommended for those traveling to Southeast Asia, persons who work closely with wild rodents in plague areas, and laboratory personnel working with *Yersinia pestis* organisms.
Pneumococcal vaccine, polyvalent	Should not be given to children under age 2 or to pregnant women.	None.	Vaccine is effective against the 23 most prevalent types of pneumococci. Administered to those who have an increased risk of developing pneumococcal pneumonia. Included are those who have chronic diseases, have had a splenectomy, are in chronic care

Table continued on following page

Name	Age Administered	Booster Schedule	Comments
			facilities or are 65 years of age or older.
Polio (inactivated poliovirus vaccine [IPV]), trivalent vaccine	At 2 and 4 months.	At 4–6 months or 11–12 years.	Administration is postponed in those with persistent vomiting, diarrhea, acute illness, or immunosuppression and in those who live in the same household as an immunosuppressed person. An alternative polio vaccine is available for immunosuppressed children.
Live oral trivalent vaccine	At 6–18 months and 4–6 years		
Rabies	See Comments.	See Comments.	Each exposure to rabies needs to be evaluated on an individual basis by the physician. Postexposure prophylaxis includes the human diploid cell vaccine and rabies immune globulin.
Typhoid	See Comments.	See Comments.	Immunization is indicated when a person

Table continued on following page

Name	Age Administered	Booster Schedule	Comments
			has come into contact with a known typhoid carrier, if there is an outbreak of typhoid fever, or prior to traveling to an area where typhoid is endemic.
Varicella zoster (chickenpox)	12–18 months.	None.	Immunizes against chickenpox in adulthood as well as childhood. The illness is much more serious in adults than in children.
Yellow fever	See Comments.	Every 10 years.	Vaccine should be given to all persons traveling or living in areas where yellow fever is present.

Source: Adapted from Taber's Cyclopedic Medical Dictionary, ed 18. FA Davis, Philadelphia, 1997, pp 2051–2053, with permission; and National Immunization Program (Centers for Disease Control and Prevention: http://www.cdc.gov/mp/announce/enhd-senequie-pr.nun) January 27, 2000.

Pediatric Developmental Milestones

Newborn: Should fixate with eyes on objects
    Equal movements
    Responds to noises

2 months: Should hold head up 45 degrees when prone
    Social smile
    Coos

4 months: Lifts head 90 degrees when prone
    Squeals
    Holds head erect when sitting
    Grasps object
    Follows object 180 degrees

6 months: Rolls over to stomach and back
    Reaches for object
    Can sit for few seconds without support

9 months: Looks for fallen object
    Feeds self a cracker
    Sits alone

    Transfers object
    Stands holding on

10 months: Pulls self to standing
    Plays peek-a-boo
    Says one word

12 months: Cruises

12–18 months: Walks
    Indicates wants without crying
    Drinks from a cup

18–24 months: Walks backward
    Feeds self with spoon
    Scribbles

24 months: Runs
    Climbs steps
    Draws a vertical line
    Solitary play

3 years: Knows first name, age
    Uses plurals in speech
    Draws a circle
    Parallel or interactive play
    Dresses with help

4 years: Knows last name
    Separates from parents

Source: Adapted from Nelms, B, and Mullins, R: Growth and Development—A Primary Care Approach. Prentice-Hall, Englewood Cliffs, NJ, 1982, pp 780–781, with permission.

Walks downstairs, both feet
alternating
Interactive games
5 years: Dresses alone
Draws a square
Follows commands
Recognizes colors

6–8 years: Skips or rollerskates
Prints numbers, letters
Can tie a bow
Defines six words
8+ years: School grade is appropriate for age

P P E N D I X

APPENDIX J

Sample of Community Resources Available for Older People

A. IN-HOME SERVICES

Meals on Wheels
Chore services (housekeeping, yardwork)
Lifeline (emergency response systems)
Home health care, equipment, supplies, wheelchairs
Transportation (medical and social)
Insurance and Medicare information
Guardianship (limited or full)
Benefits counseling (representative payee, bill paying)
Adult protective services
In-home assessment (general, medical, mental)
Care coordination (case management)
Chronic disease–related agencies (arthritic, cancer, cardiovascular disease)
Hospice services

B. RESIDENTIAL LIVING

Retirement centers
Assisted living facilities
Personal care homes
Foster home care
Shared living
Life care settings (from independent apartments to skilled nursing care)

C. INSTITUTIONAL AND HEALTH AND/OR MEDICAL RESOURCES

Nursing facilities (skilled nursing facilities, subacute care)

Hospitals (rehabilitation hospitals and units, skilled nursing units)

Long-term-care ombudsman program (advocacy for older persons)

Geriatric assessment and planning programs

Geriatric medical care (geriatrician and/or geriatric psychiatrist)

Gerontology specialists in medicine, nursing, social work, psychology

D. FAMILY SUPPORT

Widowed persons' support groups

As People Grow Older (APGO)

Children of Aging Parents support groups

Alzheimer's Association (information and support)

Adult day services

Respite care (short time)

Refer to the area agency on aging in your community for specific phone numbers and other information.

APPENDIX

Sample Cultural Assessment Guide

PERSONAL

Primary language _____ Speaks English   Yes _____ No _____

Time orientation _____

Territoriality and personal space _____

Touch permitted?   Yes _____   No _____

Physical examination permitted?   Yes _____   No _____

By whom _____

Specific requirements _____

Personal belongings _____

Other _____

DIET

Ethnic preferences _____

Religious preferences and prohibitions _____

Source: Ruff, CC, and Bloch, B: Sociocultural and spiritual dimensions of health. In Berger, KJ, and Williams, MB (eds): Fundamentals of Nursing: Collaborating for Optimal Health. Appleton & Lange, Norwalk, CT, 1992, p 239, with permission.

Diet modifications due to illness _____

Likes and dislikes _____

RELIGION

Affiliation _____

Level of participation _____

Baptism required in illness _____ Type _____

By whom _____

Rituals necessary in illness _____

Religious symbols used _____

Religious leaders _____ Role in illness _____

Medications acceptable _____

Blood transfusions acceptable   Yes _____ No _____

Special rituals _____

Other requirements _____

Omissions required _____

Do family health practices conflict with current medical practices?

   If so, how? _____

HEALTH BELIEFS AND PRACTICES

Health/illness beliefs _____

Beliefs about cause of illness _____

Traditional (folk) treatments used _____

Where obtained _____

How prepared _____

Traditional (cultural or spiritual) practitioner _____

Family caregiver _____

Treatments used _____

Beliefs about amputations, circumcision, autopsy, abortion,

euthanasia, organ donation _____

DEATH AND DYING BELIEFS AND PRACTICES

Dominant practices _____

Who should be called _____

Last rites _____

Family members' role _____

Special rituals required _____

Preparation for burial _____

Rituals regarding death _____

Who performs rituals or rites _____

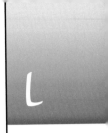

Common Disorders of Aging Minorities

African Americans. Higher incidence of strokes, obesity, cancer, glaucoma, diabetes, and hypertension than nonminority. Higher rates of chronic disease, functional impairment, and risk factors such as unemployment, poverty, and lack of adequate health care.

Native Americans. Ten times more likely to have diabetes than white people. Alcohol is the leading cause of health problems, including accidents, cirrhosis of the liver, suicide, and homicide.

Asian Americans and Pacific Islanders. Cancer is a frequent problem. Japanese Americans have a high incidence of stomach cancer. Hawaiians have a high incidence of lung and breast cancer. Chinese American women have excessive rates of pancreatic cancer. Tuberculosis also is a major concern.

Latin Americans. Higher rates of hypertension, cancer, diabetes, arthritis, and high cholesterol. High rate of chronic ailments and limitation in ADL. Have more days per year in bed because of illness.

Source: Adapted from Harper, M: Aging minorities. Healthcare Trends and Transition 6(4):17, 1995.

Sample Adult Physical Assessment Form with Guide

Name _____ Date _____

Age _____ Height/length _____ Weight _____ FOC _____

Vital Signs: T _____ P _____ R _____

BP: Sitting _____ Standing _____ Lying _____

Examination	Description*	Not Examined
Overall appearance		
Skin		
Head		

*See pp 385–391.

Source: Adapted from Physical Assessment Form 584, Harris College of Nursing, Texas Christian University, Fort Worth, TX, 2000, with permission.

Examination	Description*	Not Examined
Eyes		
Ears		
Nose and sinuses		
Mouth and pharynx		
Neck		
Thorax and lungs		
Breasts and axillae		
Heart and peripheral vascular system		
Abdomen		
Musculoskeletal system		

Genitourinary system and rectum

_____

_____

Neurologic

_____

_____

Mental status

_____

_____

Laboratory and other pertinent data

_____

_____

PHYSICAL ASSESSMENT GUIDE
General Instructions

Use this guide for suggested descriptive terminology for documentation on the Sample Adult Physical Assessment Form.

Be specific, descriptive, and objective. Avoid such terms as "normal," "within normal limits," "good," "fair," "O.K.," and so forth. Describe what you observe rather than make inferences or judgments.

Overall Appearance Inspection

Gender: Male/female.

General grooming: Clean? hair combed? makeup?

Position/posturing: Supine? prone? rigid? opisthotonos? erect? slumped?

Body size: Thin? overweight? obese? emaciated? flabby? weight proportionate to height? mesomorph? endomorph? ectomorph?

Facial expressions: Smiling? frowning? blank? apathetic?

Body language: Eye contact? no eye contact? arms folded over chest?

Other observations: Restless? fidgeting? lying quietly? listless? trembling? tense?

Skin Inspection and Palpation

Color and vascularity: Pink? tan? brown? dark brown? grayish? pasty? yellowish? flushed? jaundiced?

Turgor and mobility: Elastic? nonelastic? tenting? wrinkled? edematous? tight?

Temperature and moisture: Cold? cool? warm? hot? feverish? moist? dry? clammy? oily? sweating? diaphoresis?

Texture: Smooth? rough? fine? thick? coarse? scaly? puffy?

Nails: Clean? manicured? smooth? rough? dry? hard? brittle? splitting? cracking? angle of nail bed? clubbing? curved? flat? thick? yellowing? paronychia? *Nail beds and lunule:* Pale? pink? cyanotic? red? shape of lunule? blanching? spooning?

Body hair growth: Color? thick? thin? coarse? fine? location and distribution on body? hirsutism?

Skin integrity: Intact? not intact? *Lesions, birthmarks, moles, scars and rashes* (describe shape, size, and location): Nevi? fissures? maculas? papules? pustules? nodules? bullae? cysts? carbuncle? wheals? erythema? excoriation? desquamation? abrasions? cherry angiomas? lentigines? purpura? keratoses? seborrheic keratoses? bruises? insect bites? crusts? warts? pimples? blackheads? bleeding? drainage? lacerations? scaly? ulcers? lichenification?

Head Inspection and Palpation

Shape: Round? oval? square? pointed? normocephalic?

Face: Oval? heart-shaped? pear? long, square? round? thin? high cheekbones? symmetrical?

Sensation (trigeminal CN V): Sensation on three branches? clenched teeth?

Facial CN VII: Facial expressions, smiles?

Hair: Color and growth: coarse? fine? thick? thin? sparse? alopecia? long? short? curly? straight? permed? glossy? shiny? greasy? dry? brittle? stringy? frizzy?

Condition of scalp: Clean? scaly? dandruff? rashes? sores? drainage? Masses and lumps: Describe location and shape; measure size.

Eyes Inspection and Palpation

Eyebrows: Color and shape: Alignment? straight? curved? thick? thin? sparse? plucked? scaly?

Eyelashes: Long? short? curved? none? artificial?

Eyelids: Dark? swollen? inflamed? red? stye? infected? open and close simultaneously? ptosis? entropion? ectropion? lid lag? xanthomas?

Shape and appearance of eyes: Almond? rounded? squinty? prominent? exophthalmic? sunken? symmetrical? bright? clear? dull? tearing? discharge? (serous? purulent?) exotropia? esotropia? nystagmus? strabismus?

Sclera: White? cream? yellowish? jaundiced? injected? pterygium?

Conjunctivae: Pale pink? pink? red? inflamed? nodules? swelling?

Iris: Color and shape: Round? not round? coloboma? arcus senilis?

Cornea: Clear? milky? opaque? cloudy?

Pupils (oculomotor—CN III) [PERRLA]: Size and shape: (Measure in millimeters) Round? not round? (describe) *Equality:* Symmetrical? anisocoria? right larger than left? left larger than right? convergence? Reaction to light and accommodation? consensual reaction?

Extraocular movements (oculomotor), trochlear, abducens—CN III, IV, VI): Intact?

Lacrimal glands: Tender? nontender? inflamed? swollen? tearing?

AIDS: Glasses? contact lenses? prosthesis?

Visual fields (optic—CN II): Intact?

Vision (optic—CN II): Reads newsprint? reports objects across room?

Ears Inspection and Palpation

Pinnae: Size and shape: large? small? in proportion to face? protruding? oval? large lobes? small lobes? symmetrical? right larger than left? left larger than right? pinnae irregular? color? skin intact? redness? swelling? tophi? cauliflower ear? furuncles? Darwin's tubercle?

Level in relation to eyes: Top of pinnae level with outer canthus of eyes? top of pinnae lower than outer canthus of eyes? top of pinnae higher than outer canthus of eyes? *Canal:* Clean? discharge? (serous? bloody? purulent?) nodules? inflammation? redness? foreign object? *Cilia:* Present/absent? *Cerumen:* Present/absent? color? consistency?

Tympanic membrane: Color? pearly white? injected? red? inflamed? discharge? cone of light? landmarks? scarring? bubbles? fluid level?

Hearing (auditory—CN VII): Right—present/absent? left—present/absent? hears watch tick? hears whisper? responds readily when spoken to? *Weber:* Lateralizes equally? to left/right side? *Rinne:* Air conduction > bone conduction 2 : 1? Hearing aid: Right/left.

Nose and Sinuses Inspection and Palpation

Size and shape: Long? short? large? small? in proportion to face? flat? broad? broad based? thick? enlarged? nares symmetrical/asymmetrical? pointed? swollen? bulbous? flaring of nostrils?

Septum: Midline? deviated right/left? perforated?

Nasal mucosa and turbinates: Pink? pale? bluish? red? dry? moist? discharge? (purulent? clear? watery? mucus?) cilia present/absent? rhinnitis? epistaxis? polyps?

Patency of nares: (close each side and ask client to breathe) Right—patent/partial obstruction/obstructed? left—patent/partial obstruction/obstructed?

Olfactory (CN I): Correctly identifies odors?
Sinuses: Tender? nontender? transillumination?

Mouth and Pharynx Inspection

Lips: Color: Pink? red? tan? pale? cyanotic? *Shape:* Thin? thick? enlarged? swollen? symmetrical/asymmetrical? drooping left side? drooping right side? *Condition:* Soft? smooth? dry? cracked? fissured? blisters? lesions? (describe)

Teeth: Color and condition: White? yellow? grayish? spotted? stained? darkened? pitting? notched? straight? crooked, protruding? separated? crowded? irregular? broken? notching? peglike? loose? dull? bright? edentulous? malocclusion? *Caries and filings:* Number and location? *Dental hygiene:* Clean? not clean?

Breath odor: Sweet? odorless? halitosis? musty? acetone? foul? fetid? odor of drugs or food? hot? sour? alcohol?

Gums: Pink? firm? swollen? bleeding? sensitive? gingivitis? hypertrophy? nodules? irritated? receding? moist? ulcerated? dry? shrunken? blistered? spongy?

Facial and glossopharyngeal (CN VII and IX): Identifies taste?

Tongue: Macroglossia? microglossia? glossitis? geographic? red? pink? pale? bluish? brownish? swollen? clean? thin? thick? fissured? raw? coated? moist? dry? cracked? glistening? papillae?

Hypoglossal (CN XII): Tongue movement: symmetry? lateral? fasciculation?

Mucosa: Color? leukoplakia? dry? moist? intact? not intact? masses? (describe size, shape, and location) chancre?

Palate: Moist? dry? color? intact? not intact?

Uvula: Color? midline? Remains at midline when saying "ah"? gag reflex present?

Pharynx: Color? petechia? injected? beefy? dysphagia?

Tonsils: Present/absent? cryptic? beefy? size 1+ to 4+?

Temporomandibular joint: Fully mobile? symmetrical? tenderness? crepitus?

Neck Inspection and Palpation

Appearance: Long? short? thick? thin? masses? (describe size and shape) symmetrical? not symmetrical?

Thyroid: Palpable? nodules? tender?

Trachea: Midline? deviated to right/left?

Lymph nodes: (Occipital, preauricular, postauricular, submental, submaxillary, tonsilar, anterior cervical, posterior cervical, superficial cervical, deep cervical, supraclavicular): Nonpalpable? tender? lymphadenopathy? shotty? hard? firm?

Thorax and Lungs Inspection, Palpation, Percussion, and Auscultation

Respirations: Rate? tachypnea, eupnea, bradypnea? apnea? orthopnea? labored? stertorous? *Rhythm:* Regular/irregular? inspiration time greater than expiration time? expiration time greater than inspiration time? spasmodic? gasping? orthopneic? deep? eupneic? shallow? flaring of nostrils with respirations? symmetrical/asymmetrical? right thorax greater than left? left thorax greater than right? ratio of AP diameter to lateral diameter between 1 : 2 and 5 : 7? ribs sloped downward at 45-degree angle? well-defined costal space? accessory muscles used? pigeon chest? funnel chest? barrel chest? abdominal or chest breather? skin intact? lesions? color? thin? muscular? flabby?

Posterior thorax: Tenderness? masses? *Respiratory excursion:* Symmetrical? asymmetrical? no respiratory movements on right/left? subcutaneous emphysema? crepitus? fremitus? estimation of level of diaphragm? spine alignment? tenderness? CVA tenderness? resonance? dull? hyperresonance? diaphragmatic excursion 3 to 5 cm? comparison of one side to the other? suprasternal notch located? costochondral junctions tender? chest wall stable? vocal fremitus?

Lung auscultation: Vesicular? bronchovesicular? bronchial? whispered pectroliloquy? adventitious sounds? rales? rhonchi? wheezes? crackles? rub? bronchophony? egophony?

Breasts and Axillae Inspection and Palpation

Breasts: Male? female? present/absent? color? large? small? well developed? firm? pendulous? flat? flabby? symmetrical/asymmetrical? dimpling? thickening? smooth? retraction? peau d'orange? venous pattern? tenderness? masses? (describe) gynecomastia?

Nipples: Present/absent? circular? symmetrical/asymmetrical? inverted? everted? pale? brown? rose? extra nipples? discharge? deviation? supernumerary?

Axilla: Shaved/unshaved? odor? masses or lumps? (describe size and shape)

Lymph nodes: (Lateral, central, subscapular, pectoral, epitrochlear) palpable? tender? shotty?

Heart and Peripheral Vascular Inspection, Percussion, Auscultation, and Palpation

Heart: Precordial bulge? abnormal palpations? Point of maximum intensity? thrills? heave or lift with pulsation? S_1 loudest at apex? S_2 loudest at base? S_3? S_4? splits? clicks? snap? rub? gallop? *Murmurs:* Systolic? diastolic? holosystolic? harsh? soft? blowing?

389

...g? grading 1 through 6? high pitch? medium pitch? low
...? radiating?

Carotid pulse: Note: *Do not check both right and left carotid pulses
simultaneously. Volume:* Bounding? forceful? strong? full? weak?
feeble? thready? symmetrical? right less than left? left less than
right? *Rhythm:* Regular? irregular? symmetrical? asymmetrical?
bruits present? absent?

Apical pulse: Record rate; tachycardia? bradycardia/pounding? forceful? weak? moderate? regular/irregular?

Peripheral pulses: (Do not count rate of these pulses except radial.)
Record character, volume, rhythm, and symmetry of brachial, radial, femoral, popliteal, dorsalis pedis, and posterior tibial
pulses. *Volume:* Full? strong? forceful? bounding? perceptible?
imperceptible? weak? thready? symmetrical/asymmetrical? right
greater than left? left greater than right? *Rhythm:* Regular? irregular? symmetrical? asymmetrical? *Symmetry:* Record as symmetrical, right greater than left or left greater than right? Pulse
deficit, pulse pressure, BP in both arms, BP lying, sitting, and
standing if applicable. Jugular venous distention? (Record centimeters above level of sternal angle.)

Abdomen Inspection, Auscultation, Percussion, Palpation

Contour: Irregular? protruding? enlarged? distended? scaphoid? con-
cave? sunken? flabby? firm? flat? flaccid?

Skin: Color; intact? not intact? shiny? smooth? scars? lesions? (describe size, shape, and type of lesion) striae? umbilicus?

Bowel sounds: Present? absent? hyperactive? high-pitched tinkling?
gurgles? borborygmus?

Percussion: Tympanic? dull? flat? (describe where) liver size 6 to
12 cm? splenic dullness 6th to 10th rib? ascites?

Palpation: Splenomegaly? hepatomegaly? organomegaly? masses? aortic pulse? diastasis recti? tenderness? bulges? lower pole of kidneys
palpable? inguinal or femoral hernia? inguinal nodes? (describe)

Musculoskeletal Inspection and Palpation

Back: Shoulders level? right shoulder higher than left? left shoulder
higher than right? alignment? lordosis? scoliosis? kyphosis?
ankylosis?

Vertebral column alignment: Straight? lordosis? scoliosis? kyphosis?

Joints: Redness? swelling? deformity? (describe) crepitation? size?
symmetry? subluxation? separation? bogginess? tenderness?
pain? thickening? nodules? fluid? bulging?

Range of motion: Describe as full, limited, or fixed; estimate degree
of limitation; assess range of motion of neck, shoulders, elbows,
wrists, fingers, back, hips, knees, ankles, toes.

Extremities: Compare extremities with each other; describe color and symmetry. *Temperature:* hot, warm, cool, cold, moist, clammy, dry. Muscle tone descriptors are firm, muscular, flabby, flaccid, atrophy? fasciculation? tremor?

Lower extremities: Symmetry? (Describe any variations from normal.) abrasions? bruises? swollen? edema? rashes/lesions? (describe) prosthesis? varicose veins?

Genitourinary and Rectum Inspection

Rectum: Hemorrhoids? inflammation? lesions? skin tags? fissures? excoriation? swelling? mucosal bulging? retrocele?

Female genitalia: Pubic hair distribution and color? nits? pediculosis? lesions? nodules? inflammation? swelling? pigmentation? dry? moist? shriveled, atrophied or full labia? discharge? (describe) odor? asymmetry? varicosities? uterine prolapse? smegma? rash?

Male genitalia: Pubic hair distribution and color? nits? pediculosis? circumcised? uncircumcised? phimosis? epispadias? hypospadias? smegma? priapism? varicocele? cryptorchism, hydrocele? swelling? redness? chancre? crusting? rash? discharge? (describe) edema? scrotal sack rugated? atrophy?

Neurologic

Describe tics, twitches, paresthesia, paralysis, coordination.

Gait: Balanced? shuffling? unsteady? ataxic? parkinsonian? swaying? scissor? spastic? waddling? staggering? faltering? swaying? slow? difficult? tottering? propulsive?

Accessory—CN XI: Shrugs shoulder? symmetry?

Reflexes: Report as present or absent.

Coordination: Report as to test done.

Cranial nerves: May be reported here.

Mental Status

Level of alertness: Alert? stuporous? semicomatose? comatose?

Orientation: Oriented to time, place, and person? confused? disoriented? If confused, check orientation as follows.

Time: Ask client year, month, day, date.

Place: Ask client's residence address, where she or he is now.

Person: Ask client's name, birthday.

Memory: Recent memory: Give client short series of numbers and ask client to repeat those numbers later. *Long-term:* Ask client to recall some event that happened several years ago.

Language and speech: Language spoken? *Speech:* Slurred? slow? rapid? difficulty forming words? aphasia?

Responsiveness: Responds appropriately to verbal stimuli? responds readily? slow to respond?

Seven Warning Signs of Cancer

See your health-care provider right away if you have:

- A sore that does not get better
- A nagging cough, or unusually hoarse voice
- Indigestion (very bad upset stomach more than once in a while) or problems with swallowing
- Changes in a wart or mole
- Unusual bleeding or discharge
- Thick spot or lump in breast or anywhere else
- Change in bowel or bladder habits

Source: American Cancer Society, Inc, 1994.

Suggested Schedule of Health Screening for People Age 65 and Older with No Symptoms

SUGGESTED SCHEDULE OF HEALTH SCREENING FOR PERSONS AGE 65 AND OLDER WITH NO SYMPTOMS[1]

Exam	Both	Men	Women
1. Complete history and physical examination (including height and weight)	Annually		
2. BP; pulse (<130/85 mm Hg; 50–100 beats per minute)	Every visit with physician		
3. Urinalysis	Periodic		
4. Breast physical examination (> age 40)			Annually
5. Mammogram (> age 40)[2]			Annually
6. Pelvic examination (> age 40)			Annually
7. Pap smear[3] (> age 40)			Annually

Table continued on following page

Exam	Both	Men	Women
8. Digital rectal examination (> age 40)[2]	Annually	Check prostate annually	
9. Prostate-specific antigen (PSA) blood test (> age 50)[2]		Annually	
10. Fecal occult blood test (> age 50)[4]	Annually		
11. Dental and oral examination	Semiannually		
12. Vision exam (glaucoma,[6] cataracts)[4]	Annually		
13. Hearing examination	Periodic		
14. Total skin self-examination	Monthly		
15. Breast self-examination (BSE)			Monthly
16. Testicular self-examination (TSE)		Monthly	
17. Influenza vaccination[2]	Annually (October/ November)		
18. Pneumonia vaccination[4]	Once only (more often if high risk)		
19. Tetanus-diphtheria booster (Td)	Every 10 years after first series		
20. Hepatitis B vaccination[4,5]	Three doses— once only		
21. Tuberculosis skin test (PPD)[5]	As needed (e.g., living in nursing facility)		

Exam	Both	Men	Women
22. Cholesterol[5,6] <200 mg/dL HDL > 35 mg/dL, LDL < 130 mg/dL	Every 6 months–1 year if > 200 mg/dL		
23. Thyroid function test	Annually		
24. Blood sugar (60–110 mg/dL)[7,8]	Periodic		
25. Hematocrit/hemoglobin	Periodic		
26. Sigmoidoscopy or barium enema (> age 50)[8]	Every 2–4 years		
27. Colonoscopy or barium enema[5,6,9]	Every 2–5 years Periodic		
28. Electrocardiogram[5,6]			
29. Endometrial tissue biopsy[5]			At menopause
30. Pelvic sonogram[5]			Periodic
31. Bone mineral density (BMD) measurements (> age 50) (osteoporosis)[4–6]			Periodic
32. Chest x-ray	Not routinely recommended		

[1]These suggestions assume that the persons are healthy and not high risk (except where indicated) for any major diseases because of family history or other factors. *Individual decisions must be made by the person and physician.* Numerical norms may vary based on different references.

[2]Covered by Medicare every year.

[3]Covered by Medicare once every 3 years on an individual high-risk basis. Every year if high risk.

[4]Covered by Medicare.

[5]If high risk.

[6]Based on family history.

[7]May be higher without a diagnosis of diabetes in older adults.

[8]Covered by Medicare every 4 years.

[9]Covered by Medicare every 2 years if high risk.

REFERENCES

American Lung Association, State Office. August 10, 1994.

Barbacia, JS: Prevention. In Longergan, ET: Geriatrics. Appleton and Lange, Stamford, CT, 1996.

Crowley, SL: New Budget Finances Preventive Care. AARP Bulletin, 38(9):6, October 1997.

Cancer Facts and Figures—1994. American Cancer Society, Atlanta, GA, 1994.

Goldberg, T, and Chavm, S: Preventive Medicine and Screening in Older Adults. J Am Geriatr Soc 45:344–354, 1997.

Ham, RJ, and Sloane, PD: Primary Care Geriatrics: A Case-based Approach, ed 2. St Louis, Mosby, 1992.

Knebl, JA: Chief, Division of Geriatrics, University of North Texas Health Science Center at Fort Worth. Personal communication, 1994; March 18, 1999.

National Institute on Aging: Bound for Good Health, A Collection of Age Pages. Author, Washington, DC.

U.S. Department of Health and Human Services: Medicare and You 2001. Health Care Financing Administration, Pub. No. HCFA-10050, Baltimore, MD, 2000.

The ABCDs of Melanoma

A   *Asymmetry:* One half does not match the other half.

B   *Border irregularity:* The edges are ragged, notched, or blurred.

C   *Color:* The pigmentation is not uniform. Shades of tan, brown, and black are present. Dashes of red, white, and blue add to the mottled appearance.

D   *Diameter:* Greater than 6 mm (about the size of a pencil eraser). Any growth in size of a mole should be of concern.

Some additional warning signs of melanoma would include changes in the surface of a mole: scaliness, oozing, bleeding, or the appearance of a bump or nodule; spread of pigment from the border into surrounding skin; and change in sensation including itchiness, tenderness, or pain.

Source: American Cancer Society, 1986.

Food Guide Pyramid

A GUIDE TO DAILY FOOD CHOICES

The Food Guide Pyramid is not a prescription but a general guide of what to eat each day. It suggests eating a variety of foods to get the nutrients you need and also eating the right amounts of each food group to maintain a healthy weight. The Food Guide Pyramid emphasizes foods from the five food groups shown in the sections of the pyramid. None of these groups is more important than another; a healthy diet needs all of the nonfat groups. The Food Guide Pyramid has been modified for people age 70 and older.

These pyramids are shown on page 402.

Original Food Guide Pyramid

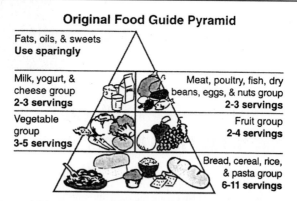

Fats, oils, & sweets
Use sparingly

Milk, yogurt, & cheese group
2-3 servings

Meat, poultry, fish, dry beans, eggs, & nuts group
2-3 servings

Vegetable group
3-5 servings

Fruit group
2-4 servings

Bread, cereal, rice, & pasta group
6-11 servings

Source: US Departments of Agriculture and Health and Human Services.

Modified Food Guide Pyramid for 70+ Adults

Fats, Oils and Sweets
USE SPARINGLY

Calcium, vitamin D, vitamin B-12
SUPPLEMENTS*

Meat, Poultry, Fish, Dry Beans, Eggs and Nut Group
≥ 2 SERVINGS

Milk, Yogurt and Cheese Group
≥ 3 SERVINGS**

Fruit Group
≥ 2 SERVINGS

Vegetable Group
≥ 3 SERVINGS

Bread, Fortified Cereal, Rice, and Pasta Group
≥ 6 SERVINGS

Water Equivalents
≥ 8 SERVINGS

● **Fat** (naturally occuring and added) © Copyright 1999 Tufts University
▼ **Sugars** (added)
f+ **Fiber** (should be present)
These symbols show fat, added sugars, and fiber in foods
*Not all individuals need supplements, consult your healthcare provider
**≥ Greater than or equal to

Source: Russell, RM, Rasmussen, H, and Lichtenstein, AH: Modified food guide pyramid for people over seventy years of age. Journal of Nutrition 129:752. © 1999 Tufts University, with permission.

Height, Weight, and Body Mass Index (BMI)

1983 METROPOLITAN HEIGHT AND WEIGHT TABLES FOR MEN AND WOMEN ACCORDING TO FRAME, AGES 25–59

Men

| Height (in shoes)* | | Weight in Pounds (in indoor clothing)† | | |
Ft	In	Small Frame	Medium Frame	Large Frame
5	2	128–134	131–141	138–150
5	3	130–136	133–143	140–153
5	4	132–138	135–145	142–156
5	5	134–140	137–148	144–160
5	6	136–142	139–151	146–164
5	7	138–145	142–154	149–168

Women

| Height (in shoes)* | | Weight in Pounds (in indoor clothing)† | | |
Ft	In	Small Frame	Medium Frame	Large Frame
4	10	102–111	109–121	118–131
4	11	103–113	111–123	120–134
5	0	104–115	113–126	122–137
5	1	106–118	115–129	125–140
5	2	108–121	118–132	128–143
5	3	111–124	121–135	131–147

ft	in	Small frame	Medium frame	Large frame
5	4	114–127	124–138	134–151
5	5	117–130	127–141	137–155
5	6	120–133	130–144	140–159
5	7	123–136	133–147	143–163
5	8	126–139	136–150	146–167
5	9	129–142	139–153	149–170
5	10	132–145	142–156	152–173
5	11	135–148	145–159	155–176
6	0	138–151	148–162	158–179

ft	in	Small frame	Medium frame	Large frame
5	8	140–148	145–157	152–172
5	9	142–151	148–160	155–176
5	10	144–154	151–163	158–180
5	11	146–157	154–166	161–184
6	0	149–160	157–170	164–188
6	1	152–164	160–174	168–192
6	2	155–168	164–178	172–197
6	3	158–172	167–182	176–202
6	4	162–176	171–187	181–297

*Shoes with 1-in heels.
†Indoor clothing weighing 5 lb for men and 3 lb for women.

Source: Taber's Cyclopedic Medical Dictionary, ed 18, 1997, p 2110, with permission.

CALCULATION OF BODY MASS INDEX

WEIGHT HEIGHT	100	105	110	115	120	125	130	135	140	145	150	155	160	165	170	175	180	185	190	195	200	205	210
5'0"	20	21	21	22	23	24	25	26	27	28	29	30	31	32	33	34	35	36	37	38	39	40	41
5'1"	19	20	21	22	23	24	25	26	26	27	28	29	30	31	32	33	34	35	36	37	38	39	40
5'2"	18	19	20	21	22	23	24	25	26	27	27	28	29	30	31	32	33	34	35	36	37	37	38
5'3"	18	19	19	20	21	22	23	24	25	26	27	27	28	29	30	31	32	33	34	35	35	36	37
5'4"	17	18	19	20	21	21	22	23	24	25	26	27	27	28	29	30	31	32	33	33	34	35	36
5'5"	17	17	18	19	20	21	22	22	23	24	25	26	27	27	28	29	30	31	32	32	33	34	35
5'6"	16	17	18	19	19	20	21	22	23	23	24	25	26	27	27	28	29	30	31	31	32	33	34
5'7"	16	16	17	18	19	20	20	21	22	23	23	24	25	26	27	27	28	29	30	31	31	32	33
5'8"	15	16	17	17	18	19	20	21	21	22	23	24	24	25	26	27	27	28	29	30	30	31	32
5'9"	15	16	16	17	18	18	19	20	21	21	22	23	24	24	25	26	27	27	28	29	30	30	31
5'10"	14	15	16	16	17	18	19	19	20	21	22	22	23	24	24	25	26	27	27	28	29	29	30
5'11"	14	15	15	16	17	17	18	19	20	20	21	22	22	23	24	24	25	26	26	27	28	29	29
6'0"	14	14	15	16	16	17	18	18	19	20	20	21	22	22	23	24	24	25	26	26	27	28	28
6'1"	13	14	15	15	16	16	17	18	18	19	20	20	21	22	22	23	24	24	25	26	26	27	28
6'2"	13	13	14	15	15	16	17	17	18	19	19	20	21	21	22	22	23	24	25	25	26	26	27
6'3"	12	13	14	14	15	16	16	17	17	18	19	19	20	21	21	22	22	23	24	24	25	26	26
6'4"	12	13	13	14	14	15	15	16	16	17	18	18	19	19	20	21	21	22	23	23	24	24	25

Here is a shortcut method for calculating BMI
(if you are too short or too tall for the table)
Example: for a person who is 5 feet 5 inches tall weighing 149 lbs.

Step 1) Multiply weight (in pounds) by 703 $149 \times 703 = 104747$

Step 2) Multiply height (in inches) by height (in inches) $65 \times 65 = 4225$

Step 3) Divide the answer in step 1 by the answer
in step 2 to get your BMI !!   104747 divided by 4225 = 24.8

BMI = 25 (rounded off)

BMI Category	Health Risk Based Solely On BMI	Risk Adjusted for the Presence of Comorbid Conditions and/or Risk Factors
19-24	Minimal	Low
25-26	Low	Moderate
27-29	Moderate	High
30-34	High	Very High
35-39	Very High	Extremely High
40+	Extremely High	Extremely High

Sources: www.jbpub.com/hwonline; www.shapeup.org.bmi/chart.htm, with permission.

Physical Signs of Malnutrition and Deficiency State

INFANTS AND CHILDREN

Lack of subcutaneous fat
Wrinkling of skin on light stroking
Poor muscle tone
Pallor
Rough skin (toad skin)
Hemorrhage of newborn, vitamin K deficiency
Bad posture
Nasal area red and greasy

Sores at angles of mouth, cheilosis
Rapid heartbeat
Red tongue
Square head, wrists enlarged, rib beading
Vincent's angina, thrush
Serious dental abnormalities
Corneal and conjunctival changes

ADOLESCENTS AND ADULTS

Nasolabial sebaceous plugs
Sores at corners of mouth, cheilosis
Vincent's angina
Minimal changes in tongue color or texture
Red swollen lingual papillae
Glossitis
Papillary atrophy of tongue
Stomatitis
Spongy, bleeding gums
Muscle tenderness in extremities
Hyperesthesia of skin

Bilateral symmetrical dermatitis
Purpura
Dermatitis: Facial butterfly, perineal, scrotal, vulval
Thickening and pigmentation of skin over bony prominences
Nonspecific vaginitis
Follicular hyperkeratosis of extensor surfaces of extremities
Rachitic chest deformity
Anemia not responding to iron

Source: **Adapted from Committee on Medical Nutrition, National Research Council.**

Poor muscle tone
Loss of vibratory sensation
Increase or decrease of tendon
  reflexes

Fatigue of visual accommoda-
  tion
Vascularization of cornea
Conjunctival changes

OLDER ADULTS

Progressive weight loss
Reduced appetite
Prominence of the bony
  skeleton
Muscle wasting
Glossitis
Mouth sores
Cracked lips
Brittle hair and nails
Dry rough skin
Nonhealing wounds

Sunken eyes
Pale sclerae
Peripheral edema
Lack of energy or generalized
  weakness
Blunted mental status
Decreased deep tendon re-
  flexes
Decreased vibratory sense
Bleeding gums and poor den-
  tition

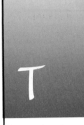
Ten Tips for Healthy Aging

1. Eat a balanced diet.
2. Exercise regularly.
3. Get regular checkups.
4. Do not smoke. It is never too late to quit.
5. Practice safety habits at home to prevent falls and fractures. Always wear your seat belt when traveling by car.
6. Maintain contacts with family and friends, and stay active through work, recreation, and community.
7. Avoid overexposure to the sun and the cold.
8. If you drink, do so in moderation. When you drink, let someone else drive.
9. Keep personal and financial records in order to simplify budgeting and investing. Plan long-term housing and financial needs.
10. Keep a positive attitude toward life. Do things that make you happy.

Source: National Institute on Aging, National Institutes of Health, Rockville, Md.

Vitamin and Mineral Dosages Recommended for Persons 65 and Older

RECOMMENDED DOSAGES: VITAMINS AND SELECTED MINERALS FOR PERSONS 65 AND OLDER

Caution: References differ on recommended and maximum doses. Food sources are best. Large doses may interfere with medications and/or herbal products. Check with physician about individual needs, doses, and precautions.

Vitamin or Mineral	Benefit	Recommended daily dose	Food sources	Maximum dose	Possible side effects with excessive doses
A (fat-soluble)	Skin, eyes, mucous membranes	5000 IU (M) 4000 IU (W) 1000 RE (M) 800 RE (W)	Liver, eggs, butter, milk, broccoli, greens, carrots, cantaloupe	Five times recommended amount	Headache, nausea, irritability, hair loss; interfere with cell growth
B_6 (water-soluble)	Brain, nerves, heart, arteries, immune system	2.0 mg (M) 1.6 mg (W)	Tuna, vegetables, banana, bran cereal	2.2 mg (M) 2 mg (W)	Nerve damage
B_{12} (water-soluble)	Blood cells, cognitive function	3 µg	Liver, milk, eggs, shrimp, pork, chicken		

Nutrient	Function	RDA	Sources	Supplement	Side Effects/Notes
C* (water-soluble)	Growth and repair of tissue, wound and bone repair, increase high-density lipids (HDL), may protect against some types of cancer, decrease cell damage	60 mg	Orange juice, tomatoes, green vegetables	250–500 mg; up to 1000 mg	
D (fat-soluble)	Bones (aids in calcium absorption)	400 IU	Sun, foods fortified with vitamin D if not exposed to sun	600–800 IU	Nausea, weight loss, excess urination, calcium deposits in organs
E* (fat-soluble)	Heart, arteries, immune system, reduce cell damage	200–400 IU 10 mg (M) 8 mg (W)	Whole grains, dark leafy vegetables, nuts, beans	800–1200 IU	Should not be taken with certain prescription medications (for example, anticoagulants)
K (fat-soluble)	Clotting of blood	80 µg (M) 65 µg (W)	Liver, spinach, broccoli		Blood clots
Calcium*	Bones, blood clotting, heart, muscles	1500 mg	Milk, cheese, yogurt, turnip greens, broccoli	1500 mg	Kidney/bladder stones if not active

Table continued on following page

413

Vitamin	Benefit	Recommended daily dose	Food sources	Maximum dose	Possible side effects with excessive doses
Potassium	Blood pressure, cellular function	3000 mg	Apricots, bananas, oranges, juice, poultry, meat	6725 mg	
Zinc	Heal wounds, immune system, taste and smell, cell division and growth	15 mg (M) 12 mg (W)	Meat, poultry, fish, beans, grains	50 mg–220 mg treatment for skin problems	
Water*	Urinary system, nutrients to all cells	Six to eight 8-oz. glasses	Preferably water and juices—also soup and gelatin; limit caffeine and alcohol	100 oz	May be contraindicated in high blood pressure, renal dialysis, and some heart conditions

KEY: IU—International units; RE—Retinol equivalents; M—Men; W—Women; mg—milligrams; μg—micrograms; μg—1 RE
*Especially important for this age group

REFERENCES

Cummings, D: Geriatric Nutrition. Tarrant Area Gerontological Society Summer Forum. Fort Worth, TX, July 13, 1999.

Insel, PM, and Walton, RT: Core Concepts in Health. Mayfield, Mountain View, CA, 1996.

Robinson, N: Dietary management. In MO Hogstel (ed), Nursing Care of the Older Adult. New York, Delmar, 1994.

Taber's Cyclopedic Medical Dictionary, ed 18. Davis, Philadelphia, 1997.

Top 100 foods. Berkeley Wellness Letter. University of California, Berkeley, 1999.

U.S. News and World Report: 1994 Family Health Almanac. Author, Washington, DC, 1994.

Van Beber, A: Food and nutrition services. In MO Hogstel (ed), Community Resources for Older Adults: A Guide for Case Managers. Mosby, St Louis, 1998.

APPENDIX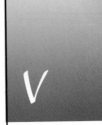

Glasgow Coma Scale

Eye Opening	Points	Best Verbal Response	Points	Best Motor Response	Points
Spontaneous: Indicates arousal mechanisms in brainstem are active.	4	*Oriented:* Patient knows who and where he is, and the year, season, and month.	5	*Obeys commands:* Do not class a grasp reflex or change in posture as a response.	6
To sound: Eyes open to any sound stimulus.	3	*Confused:* Responses to questions indicate varying degrees of confusion and disorientation.	4	*Localized:* Moves a limb to attempt to remove stimulus	5
To pain: Apply stimulus to limbs, not to face.	2	*Inappropriate:* Speech is intelligible, but sustained conversation is not possible.	3	*Flexor normal:* Entire shoulder or arm is flexed in response to painful stimuli.	4

Never	1	*Flexion abnormal:* Slow stereotyped assumption of decorticate rigidity posture in response to painful stimuli.	3
Incomprehensible: Patient makes unintelligible sounds such as moans and groans.	2	*Extension:* Abnormal with adduction and internal rotations of the shoulder and pronation of the forearm.	2
None	1	*None:* Be certain that a lack of response is not due to a spinal cord injury.	1

NOTE: This scale, originally described in 1974 and further discussed in 1979 by Teasdale and his associates, is widely used in assessing head injury patients, both at the time of the injury and as the patient is observed. The score is recorded every 2 to 3 days.

Source: Adapted from Teasdale, G, and Jennet, B: Lancet II, 1974, p 81, and Teasdale, G, et al: Acta Neurochirurgica (suppl) 28, 1979, pp 13–16.

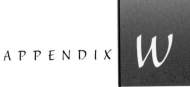

A P P E N D I X

Dermatomes

Source: Taber's Cyclopedic Medical Dictionary, ed 18. FA Davis, Philadelphia, 1997, p 520, with permission.

421

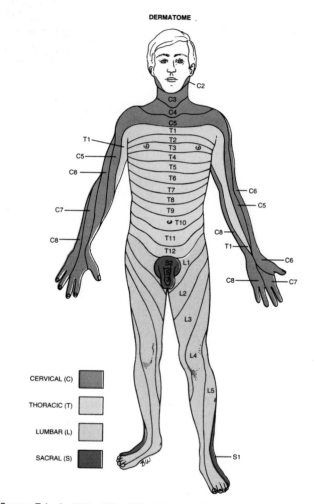

DERMATOME

Source: Taber's, 1997, ed 18, p 520, with permission.

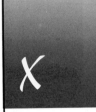

APPENDIX X

Client Positions

Source: Taber's, 1997, ed 18, pp 1528–1529, with permission.

POSITIONS

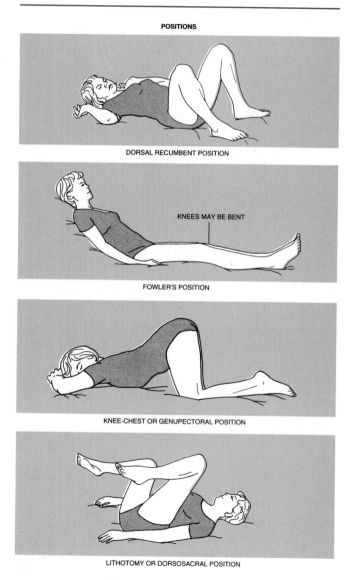

DORSAL RECUMBENT POSITION

KNEES MAY BE BENT

FOWLER'S POSITION

KNEE-CHEST OR GENUPECTORAL POSITION

LITHOTOMY OR DORSOSACRAL POSITION

POSITIONS

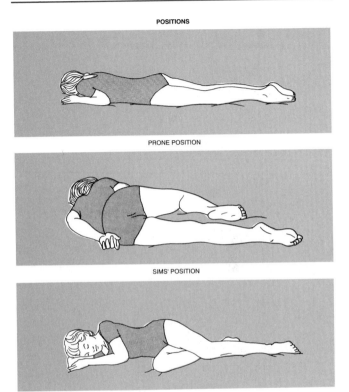

PRONE POSITION

SIMS' POSITION

RIGHT LATERAL RECUMBENT POSITION

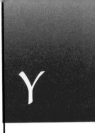

Conversion Rules

To convert units of one system into the other, multiply the number of units in column I by the equivalent factor opposite that unit in column II.

WEIGHT		
I		**II**
1 milligram	—	0.015432 grain
1 gram	—	15.432 grains
1 gram	—	0.25720 apothecaries' dram
1 gram	—	0.03527 avoirdupois ounce
1 gram	—	0.03215 apothecaries' or troy ounce
1 kilogram	—	35.274 avoirdupois ounces
1 kilogram	—	32.151 apothecaries' or troy ounces
1 kilogram	—	2.2046 avoirdupois pounds
1 grain	—	64.7989 milligrams
1 grain	—	0.0648 gram
1 apothecaries' dram	—	3.8879 grams
1 avoirdupois ounce	—	28.3495 grams
1 apothecaries' or troy ounce	—	31.1035 grams
1 avoirdupois pound	—	453.5924 grams

VOLUME (AIR OR GAS)		
I		**II**
1 cubic centimeter	—	0.06102 cubic inch
1 cubic meter	—	35.314 cubic feet

Table continued on following page

1 cubic meter	—	1.3079 cubic yard
1 cubic inch	—	16.3872 cubic centimeters
1 cubic foot	—	0.02832 cubic meter

CAPACITY (FLUID OR LIQUID)		
I		**II**
1 milliliter	—	16.23 minim
1 milliliter	—	0.2705 fluidram
1 milliliter	—	0.0338 fluidounce
1 liter	—	33.8148 fluidounces
1 liter	—	2.1134 pints
1 liter	—	1.0567 quart
1 liter	—	0.2642 gallon
1 fluidram	—	3.697 milliliters
1 fluidounce	—	29.573 milliliters
1 pint	—	473.1765 milliliters
1 quart	—	946.353 milliliters
1 gallon	—	3.785 liters

TO CONVERT CELSIUS OR CENTIGRADE DEGREES TO FAHRENHEIT DEGREES

Multiply the number of Celsius degrees by ⅕ and add 32 to the result.

Example: $55°C \times ⅘ = 99 + 32 = 131°F$

TO CONVERT FAHRENHEIT DEGREES TO CELSIUS DEGREES

Subtract 32 from the number of Fahrenheit degrees and multiply the difference by ⅝.

Example: $243°F - 32 = 211 \times ⅝ = 117.2°C$

Source: Adapted from Taber's Cyclopedic Medical Dictionary, ed 18, 1997, pp 703, 2231, with permission.

Weights and Measures

APOTHECARIES' WEIGHT

20 grains = 1 scruple
8 grains = 1 ounce

3 scruples = 1 dram
12 ounces = 1 pound

AVOIRDUPOIS WEIGHT

27.343 grains = 1 dram
16 ounces = 1 pound
2000 pounds = 1 short ton
1 oz troy = 480 grains
1 lb troy = 5760 grains

16 drams = 1 ounce
100 pounds = 1 hundredweight
2240 pounds = 1 long ton
1 oz avoirdupois = 437.5 grains
1 lb avoirdupois = 7000 grains

CIRCULAR MEASURE

60 seconds = 1 minute
90 degrees = 1 quadrant

60 minutes = 1 degree
4 quadrants = 360 degrees = circle

CUBIC MEASURE

1728 cubic inches = 1 cubic foot
2150.42 cubic inches = 1 standard bushel
1 cubic foot = about four-fifths of a bushel

27 cubic feet = 1 cubic yard
268.8 cubic inches = 1 dry (U.S.) gallon
128 cubic feet = 1 cord (wood)

DRY MEASURE

2 pints = 1 quart	8 quarts = 1 peck	4 pecks = 1 bushel

LIQUID MEASURE

16 ounces = 1 pint	4 quarts = 1 gallon	2 barrels = 1 hogshead (U.S.)
1000 milliliters = 1 liter	31.5 gallons = 1 barrel (U.S.)	1 quart = 946.35 milliliters
4 gills = 1 pint	2 pints = 1 quart	1 liter = 1.0566 quart

Barrels and hogsheads vary in size. A U.S. gallon is equal to 0.8327 British gallon; therefore, a British gallon is equal to 1.201 U.S. gallon. 1 liter is equal to 1.0567 quart.

LINEAR MEASURE

1 inch = 2.54 centimeters	40 rods = 1 furlong	8 furlongs = 1 statute mile
12 inches = 1 foot	3 feet = 1 yard	5.5 yards = 1 rod
1 statute mile = 5280 feet	3 statute miles = 1 statute league	1 nautical mile = 6076.042 feet

Table continued on following page

431

TROY WEIGHT

24 grains = 1 pennyweight   20 pennyweights = 1 ounce   12 ounces = 1 pound

Used for weighing gold, silver, and jewels

HOUSEHOLD MEASURES* AND WEIGHTS

Approximate Equivalents: 60 gtt.

= 1 teaspoonful = 5 mL = 60 minims = 60 grains = 1 dram = ⅛ ounce

1 teaspoon = ⅛ fl. oz; 1 dram   16 tablespoons (liquid) = 1 cup

3 teaspoons = 1 tablespoon   12 tablespoons (dry) = 1 cup

1 tablespoon = ½ fl. oz; 4 drams   1 cup = 8 fl. oz

1 tumbler or glass = 8 fl. oz; ½ pint

*Household measures are not precise. For instance, a household teaspoon will hold from 3 to 5 mL of liquid substances. Therefore, do not substitute household equivalents for medication prescribed by the physician.

Source: Taber's Cyclopedic Medical Dictionary, ed 18. FA Davis, Philadelphia, 1997, p 2230, with permission.

Fahrenheit and Celsius Scales

THERMOMETRIC EQUIVALENTS (CELSIUS AND FAHRENHEIT)

C°	F°	C°	F°	C°	F°	C°	F°
0	32	27	80.6	54	129.2	81	177.8
1	33.8	28	82.4	55	131	82	179.6
2	35.6	29	84.2	56	132.8	83	181.4
3	37.4	30	86.0	57	134.6	84	183.2
4	39.2	31	87.8	58	136.4	85	185
5	41	32	89.6	59	138.2	86	186.8
6	42.8	33	91.4	60	140	87	188.6
7	44.6	34	93.2	61	141.8	88	190.4
8	46.4	35	95	62	143.6	89	192.2
9	48.2	36	96.8	63	145.4	90	194
10	50	37	98.6	64	147.2	91	195.8
11	51.8	38	100.4	65	149	92	197.6
12	53.6	39	102.2	66	150.8	93	199.4
13	55.4	40	104	67	152.6	94	201.2
14	57.2	41	105.8	68	154.4	95	203
15	59	42	107.6	69	156.2	96	204.8
16	60.8	43	109.4	70	158	97	206.6
17	62.6	44	111.2	71	159.8	98	208.4
18	64.4	45	113	72	161.6	99	210.2
19	66.2	46	114.8	73	163.4	100	212
20	68	47	116.6	74	165.2		
21	69.8	48	118.4	75	167		
22	71.6	49	120.2	76	168.8		
23	73.4	50	122	77	170.6		
24	75.2	51	123.8	78	172.4		
25	77	52	125.6	79	174.2		
26	78.8	53	127.4	80	176		

Source: Taber's Cyclopedic Medical Dictionary, ed 18. FA Davis, Philadelphia, 1997, p 1939, with permission.

Medication Card

```
                MEDICATION CARD
NAME _._____

ADDRESS _____
        _____

DATE OF BIRTH _____

DATE CARD FILLED OUT _____

EMERGENCY CONTACT PHONE _____

HOSPITAL PREFERRED _____

PHYSICIAN _____
    PHONE _____

MAJOR ILLNESSES




MEDICATION ALLERGIES


```

Medication card. **Source:** Harris School of Nursing, Texas Christian University, 2000. Used with permission.

PRESCRIPTION MEDICATIONS		
NAME	DOSE	TIMES TAKEN

OVER-THE-COUNTER-MEDICATIONS		
(vitamins, herbs, supplements)		

TCU

TAKE CARE OF YOUR HEALTH
HARRIS SCHOOL OF NURSING
TEXAS CHRISTIAN UNIVERSITY

Newborn Physical Assessment Guide

This is a guide to assist you in the assessment of a newborn. The first term in the category is usually the normal expected finding, *italicized words* are variations of normal or abnormal findings, *italicized and underlined* are gestational age assessment findings.

GENERAL INFORMATION

(You may obtain this information from mother's and baby's charts) Length of prenatal care? high-risk factors? date of birth? type of delivery? pregnancy/delivery complications? birth length? Apgar scores? gestation (weeks)? age (days/hours)? today's weight? birth weight?

Skin Inspection and Palpation

Color and vascularity: Ethnic grouping? pink? acrocyanosis? Mongolian spots? milia? *central cyanosis? pale? plethoric? mottled? jaundice? abrasions? birthmarks? meconium staining? ecchymosis? lacerations? petechiae? opacity?*

Turgor: Elastic? *tenting?*

Temperature and moisture: Dry? moist?

Texture and integrity: Smooth and intact? *eruptions? not intact? lesions? pustules? rash? skin tags? vesicles? lanugo? peeling? dry?*

Nails: Soft? cover entire nail bed? beyond fingertips? meconium staining?

Head Inspection and Palpation

Shape: Symmetrical without molding? *caput? asymmetrical? molding? cephalhematoma? forceps marks?*

Fontanel: Flat? *sunken? full? bulging? tense? sagittal suture—smooth without ridges? overriding?*

Source: **Harris School of Nursing, Texas Christian University, Fort Worth, Tex, 2000, with permission.**

Face: Symmetrical? *asymmetrical?*

Eyes Inspection

Sclera: Clear? bluish-white? blink reflex? *jaundice? tearing?*
Conjunctiva: Clear? *jaundice? hemorrhage?*
Pupils: Reactions to light? PERRL
Retina: Red reflex present?
Eyelids: Movements? *prominent epicanthal folds? placement? edema?*
Eye movements: Present?

Ears Inspection and Palpation

Pinnae: Position/placement: aligned with eyes? skin tags? preauricular sinus? *curvature? cartilage development? recoil?*

Nose Inspection and Palpation

Symmetrical and midline? patency? milia? discharge?

Mouth Inspection and Palpation

Lips: Symmetrical? *thin upper lip?*
Shape:
Palates: Hard palate-intact? soft palate-intact?
Mucous membrane: Dry? pink? *cyanosis? pale? thrush? Epstein's pearls?*
Sucking reflex: Strong? *weak? uncoordinated? frantic?*
Swallow: Strong? *weak? uncoordinated?*
Tongue: Movement: *protrusion? retrusion? coating?* size and integrity: *hypertrophied?*
Uvula: Intact? midline? *bifid?*

Neck Inspection and Palpation

Movement: Full ROM? *head lag?* limited ROM?
Symmetry: Webbing? *multiple skin folds?*
Masses: *Above or lateral to clavicle?*
Trachea: Midline?
Enlarged thyroid? None palpated

Chest Inspection, Palpation, and Auscultation

Symmetry and proportion: Barrel chest? *supranummary nipples? breast discharge?* breast engorgement?

Clavicles: Straight? smooth? *crepitus R or L?*
Respirations: Rate? rhythm? thoracic or abdominal breathing? *retractions? grunting? nasal flaring? seesaw respirations?*
Breath sounds: Equal? clear? *rales? rhonchi?*

Heart and Peripheral Vascular Inspection, Palpation, and Auscultation

Heart: Rate? rhythm? murmurs? PMI? S_1? S_2?
Peripheral pulses: Present, bilateral, symmetrical? (brachial, radial, femoral, popliteal, dorsalis pedis?)
Precordium: Movement?

Abdomen Inspection, Auscultation, Palpation, and Percussion

Shape and symmetry: Rounded? symmetrical? *flat? protuberant? scaphoid? asymmetrical? distended?*
Muscle tone: Soft? *flabby and wrinkled? hard and rigid?*
Bowel sounds: Present in all four quadrants? *absent?*
Umbilical stump: Drying? *redness? discharge? bleeding?*
Umbilical vessels: 2 or 3? *meconium staining (see before dye applied)? hernia?*
Bladder distention: Absent? *present?*

Genitalia/Genitourinary Inspection and Palpation

Female: Labia? position of meatus? *vaginal discharge? hymenal tag? size of labia majora versus minora?*
Male: Penis—position of meatus? circumcision? urination within 24 hours? *epispadias? hypospadias? scrotum enlarged? hydrocele? testicles descended? scrotum-rugae?*
Anus: Location? patency? meconium?
Buttocks: Edema or bruising of buttocks?

Spine Inspection and Palpation

Closed vertebral column? alignment in prone position? incurvation of trunk? Mongolian spot? *pilonidal dimple/sinus? tuft of hair? asymmetry? mass?*

Hips Inspection and Palpation

Symmetrical or *asymmetrical* gluteal fold? *abduction angle? knee-hip length equal? Ortolani maneuver done—any click felt?*

Musculoskeletal Inspection and Palpation

Hands and Feet: Number of digits? ROM? *presence of creases? 1/3, 2/3 or complete surface of soles and palms w/creases? scarf sign? square window? arm recoil? heel to ear flexion?*

Arms and Legs: ROM? flexion? symmetry? equal movements? *positional deformities?*

Neurologic Inspection and Palpation

Reflexes: Hands-grasp reflex? plantar reflex? Babinski reflex? stepping reflex? Moro reflex? tonic neck?

Tone: Normal flexion? *flaccidity? spasticity?*

Cry: Normal? no cry, alert and quiet? *weak? shrill? hoarse?*

Behavioral (Observation)

Activity: Active? active with stimulation? quiet? sleeping? baby quiets to soothing, cuddling, or wrapping? *lethargic? irritable? tremors? excessive crying? fretfulness? unable to quiet self?*

Glossary

A "P" following a term or an abbreviation signifies that it is particularly pertinent in pediatric assessment. A "G" following a term or an abbreviation means that it is particularly pertinent in geriatric assessment. An "R" following a term or abbreviation means that it is particularly pertinent in racial and ethnic assessment.

Accommodation: The ability of the eyes to adapt to viewing objects at various distances

Acrochordons [G]: Skin tags

Acrocyanosis [P]: Blueness (cyanosis) of the newborn's hands and feet caused by slow peripheral perfusion

AC: Air conduction

ADL: Activity of daily living

Adventitious: Abnormal breath sounds

AFDC: Aid to Families with Dependent Children

AK: Above the knee

Alopecia: Loss of hair on head

Ankyloglossia [P]: Tongue-tie

A/P: Anterior/posterior

Apgar score: Screening tool for newborn at birth

Arcus senilis [G]: An opaque white ring around the periphery of the cornea (not pathologic)

Ascites: Serous fluid in abdominal cavity

AV: Arteriovenous

B/A: Bone/air in Rinne hearing test

Barlow's sign: Maneuver to detect subluxation or dislocation of the hip

BC: Bone conduction

Borborygmus: Gurgling, splashing sound over large intestines

BP: Blood pressure

BSC: Bedside commode

BSE: Breast self-examination

Brudzinski's sign [P]: Flexion of hips when neck is flexed from supine position

Bruits: Vascular sounds similar to heart murmurs that may be auscultated in areas such as the carotid artery, temple, and epigastrium

Capillary hemangioma [P]: A congenital lesion consisting of numerous closely packed capillaries separated by a network of cells

Caput succedaneum [P]: An edematous swelling of the scalp caused by pressure

CC: Chief complaint, reason that client is presenting for care or examination

Cephalhematoma [P]: A subperiosteal hemorrhage caused by birth trauma; does not cross suture lines

Cerumen: Earwax

Chloasma: Hyperpigmentation, especially of face, commonly associated with pregnancy

Clubbing: Abnormal enlargement of the distal ends of the fingers and toes, together with curvature of the nails

CN: Cranial nerve

CN I: Olfactory nerve

CN II: Optic nerve

CN III: Oculomotor nerve

CN IV: Trochlear nerve

CN V: Trigeminal nerve

CN VI: Abducens nerve

CN VII: Facial nerve

CN VIII: Acoustic nerve

CN IX: Glossopharyngeal nerve

CN X: Vagus nerve

CN XI: Spiral accessory nerve

CN XII: Hypoglossal nerve

Coloboma: A defect of the pupil of the eye (keyhole pupil)

Comedones [P]: Blackheads

Consanguinity: Related by blood

Consensual constriction: A reflex action whereby a light beam directed into one eye causes not only the pupil of that eye but also that of the other eye to constrict

Crepitus: Crackling noise similar to rubbing hair between fingers

CT scan: Computed tomography scan

C-V: Cardiovascular

CVA: Cerebrovascular accident; stroke

Cx: Cervix

Cyanosis: Blue-gray color of skin

Denver II: Developmental screening tool for children to age 6

DES: Diethylstilbestrol

Diastasis recti: Lateral separation of the two halves of the musculus rectum dominis

DOB: Date of birth

DTRs: Deep tendon reflexes

Dx: Diagnosis

Dyspnea: Difficulty breathing

Dysuria: Difficult painful urination

ECG: Electrocardiogram

Ectropion: Eversion of the edge of an eyelid

EDC: Expected date of confinement

Edema: Swelling

Encopresis: Involuntary discharge of watery feces associated with constipation and fecal retention

ENT: Ear, nose, and throat

Entropion: Inversion of the edge of an eyelid

Enuresis: Involuntary discharge of urine

EOM: Extraocular movement

Epistaxis: Nosebleed

Epstein's pearls [P]: White-yellow accumulation of epithelial cells on hard palate of newborn

Erythema: Diffused redness of skin

Erythema toxicum neonatorum [P]: A common rash in newborns, characterized by papules or pustules on an erythematous base

Excursion (respiratory): Extent of movement of the diaphragm

Exophthalmos: Abnormal protrusion of eyeball

Exudate: Accumulation of fluid, pus, or serum or matter that penetrates through vessel wall

FHT: Fetal heart tone

Fremitus: A vibration palpated or auscultated through the chest wall

G (for gravid): Pregnant

Gastroschisis [P]: Congenital opening in the wall of the abdomen

Genu valgum: Knock-knee

Genu varum: Bowleg

Gravity: The number of pregnancies

Harlequin sign [P]: A transient redness on one side of the body and paleness on the other; cause unknown

HIV: Human immunodeficiency virus

Hirsutism: Excessive growth of hair in unusual places

Hordeolum: Inflammation of a sebaceous gland of the eyelid

Hx: History

Hypertelorism: Abnormal width between two organs, for example, eyes

Hypertropia: Abnormal turning of eyes upward

Hypotropia: Abnormal turning of eyes downward

IADL: Instrumental activity of daily living

ICS: Intercostal space

Jaundice [P]: Yellowing of the skin; physiologic jaundice; mild jaundice of the newborn caused by functional immaturity of the liver, which results in yellowing after the first 24 hours

JVP: Jugular venous pressure

Keloid [R]: Increased scar formation from previous surgery and/or trauma

Kernig's sign: Reflex contraction and pain in hamstring muscles when extending the leg after flexing the thigh upon the body

Koplik's spots: Small red spots on oral mucosa (sign of measles)

Lanugo [P]: Fine downy hair on the body of infants, especially premature infants

L & W: Living and well

LCM: Left costal margin

Leukoplakia: Formation of white spots or patches on the mucous membrane of the tongue or cheek

Leukorrhea: White or yellow discharge from cervical canal or vagina

LICS: Left intercostal space

LLQ: Left lower quadrant

LMP: Last menstrual period

Lordosis, kyphosis, scoliosis: Swayback, hunchback, lateral curvature of spine

LSB: Left sternal border

LUL: Left upper lobe

LUQ: Left upper quadrant

Macule: See lesion list

MCL: Midclavicular line

Menarche: The onset of menses

Metatarsus adductus: Adduction of the forefoot distal to the metatarsal-tarsal line

Milia [P]: Obstructed sebaceous glands, frequently found on the nose and cheeks

Mongolian spot [P]: A bluish black area over the sacral areas of dark-skinned infants

Montgomery's tubercles: Lubricating glands on nipples

Morphology: The science of structure and form

MRI: Magnetic resonance imaging

MSL: Midsternal line

Nevus flammeus [P]: A circumscribed red, flat lesion found on the face, eyelid, and neck of infants

NG: Nasogastric

Nuchal: Of the neck

Nulliparous: Without births or pregnancies beyond 20 weeks' gestation

Nystagmus: Constant involuntary movement of eyeball

OD: Right eye (L, oculo dextro)

Onychomycosis [G]: A fungus infection of the nails, causing thickening, roughness, and splitting

Orthopnea: Breathing easier in erect position

Ortolani test [P]: Test for a congenitally dislocated hip in an infant

OS: Left eye (L, oculo sinistro)

OTC: Over the counter (i.e., nonprescription)

OU: Both eyes (L, oculi unitas)

Pap: Papanicolaou smear

Paresthesia: Numbness, prickling, tingling

Parity: The state of having borne an infant or infants

Peau d'orange: Dimpled skin condition that resembles the skin of an orange

Pectus carinatum: Abnormal prominence of the sternum

Pectus excavatum: Abnormal depression of the sternum

Peristalsis: Wavelike movements of the alimentary canal

PERRLA: Pupils equal, round, reactive to light and accommodation

PI: Present illness

Pinna: Auricle or exterior ear

PMI: Point of maximum intensity

Polydactyly: Abnormal number of fingers and toes

Presbycusis [G]: Decreased hearing associated with later maturity

Pseudofolliculitis [R]: Small inflamed pustules near hair follicles caused by shaving too close or short curly hairs that reenter the skin

Ptosis: Drooping of body part (e.g., eyelid)

PVC: Preventricular contraction

Rales: Crackles; added noncontinuous crackling sounds heard on auscultation of the chest; an adventitious sound

RCM: Right costal margin

Rhonchi: Gurgles; added continuous, sonorous, low-pitched sounds heard on auscultation of the chest

Rinne test: A test in which a vibrating tuning fork is used to determine whether a person has normal hearing by comparing the sound perception by bone conduction and by air conduction

RLQ: Right lower quadrant

RRR: Regular rate and rhythm

RUQ: Right upper quadrant

S_1, S_2, S_3, S_4: Heart sounds

Scaphoid: Boat-shaped, sunken

SIADH: Syndrome of inappropriate antidiuretic hormone

SIDS [P]: Sudden infant death syndrome

Snellen E chart: A wall eye chart

SPF: Skin protection factor for sunscreens and blocks

STD: Sexually transmitted disease

Strabismus: A condition in which the optic axes of the eyes cannot be directed to some object

Striae: Stretch marks, or scarlike breaks in the skin, usually caused by stretching of the skin from weight gain

Syndactyly [P]: Fusion of the toes or fingers

TDD: Telephone device for the deaf

TENS: Transcutaneous electrical nerve stimulation used to relieve pain

Thelarche [P]: Beginning of breast development at puberty

Thrills: Palpable murmur or rub

Tophi: Mineral deposits; tartar

TORCH: Toxoplasmosis, other (viruses), rubella, cytomegalovirus, herpes (simplex viruses)

Torticollis: Head tilts to one side with chin pointing to the other side

Torus palatinus: Benign bony protuberance at the midline of the hard palate

TSE: Testicular self-examination

Turgor: Elasticity of skin

TURP [G]: Transurethral resection of the prostate gland

UTI: Urinary tract infection

Vernix caseosa [P]: A white cheeselike substance found on the skin folds of newborns

Vertigo: Dizziness or lightheadedness

Vesicular: Pertaining to the alveoli of the lungs

Vitiligo: Patches of depigmented skin, piebald skin

Weber test for hearing: A test in which a vibrating tuning fork is used to determine which ear is affected by hearing loss

References

PART 1

American Association of Retired Persons and the Administration on Aging: A Profile of Older Americans: 1999. U.S. Department of Health and Human Services, 1998, pp 2, 4.

Browning, M: Home environment assessment guide. In Hogstel, M (ed): Nursing Care of the Older Adult, ed 3. Delmar, Albany, NY, 1994, pp 592–595.

Clark, JM: Nursing in the Community: Dimensions of Community Health Nursing, ed 3. Appleton and Lange, Stamford, CT, 1999.

Folstein, MF, Folstein, SE, and McHugh, PR: Mini-mental state. Journal of Psychiatric Research, 12(1):189–198, 1975.

Friedman, MM: Family Nursing Theory and Practice, ed 3. McGraw-Hill, New York, 1992.

Gallo, JJ, Reichel, W, and Andersen, LM: Handbook of Geriatric Assessment, ed 2. Aspen, Gaithersburg, MD, 1995.

Geissler, E: Quick Reference to Cultural Assessment. Mosby, St Louis, 1994.

Giger, JN, and Davidhizer, RE: Transcultural Nursing: Assessment and Intervention, ed 2. Mosby, St Louis, 1995.

Hogstel, MO: Assessing mental status. J Geront Nurs 17(5):43, 1991.

Johnson, BS, and Baggett, JM: Applying the nursing process to children, adolescents, and families. In Johnson, BS (ed): Child, Adolescent, and Family Psychiatric Nursing. Lippincott, Philadelphia, 1995.

Katz, S, Ford, AB, and Moskowitz, RW, et al: Studies of illness in the aged: The index of ADL. JAMA 185:914–919, 1963.

Long, BC, Phipps, W, and Cassmeyer, VL: Medical-Surgical Nursing: A Nursing Process Approach. Mosby, St Louis, 1994.

Mahoney, FI, and Barthel, DW: Functional evaluation: The Barthel index. Maryland Med J 14:61–65, 1965.

Seidel, HM, Ball, JW, Dains, JE, and Benedict, GW: Mosby's Guide to Physical Examination, ed 4. Mosby Year–Book, St Louis, 1999.

Sidell, M: Health in Old Age. Open University Press, Buckingham, England, 1994.

Stanhope, M, and Lancaster, J: Community Health Nursing: Promoting Health of Aggregates, Families and Individuals, ed 4. Mosby, St Louis, 1996.

PART 2

Kozier, B, Erb, G, Blais, K, Wilkinson, JM, and Van Leuven, K. (eds): Fundamentals of Nursing, ed 5. Addison-Wesley, Menlo Park, CA, 1998.

Muecke, MA: Culture and ethnicity. In Craven, RF, and Hirnle, CJ (eds): Fundamentals of Nursing: Human Health and Function. Lippincott, Philadelphia, 1992, pp 236–252.

PART 3

Cox, CR, and Bloch, B: Sociocultural and spiritual dimensions of health. In Berger, KJ, and Williams, MB: Fundamentals of Nursing Collaborating for Optimal Health. Appleton and Lange, East Norwalk, CT, 1992, pp 210–243.

Edelman, DL, and Mandle, CL: Health Promotion throughout the Lifespan, ed 4. Mosby, St Louis, 1998.

Hogstel, MO: Vital signs are really vital in the old-old. Geriatr Nurs 15(5):252–256, 1994.

Jarvis, C. (ed): Physical Examination and Health Assessment. WB Saunders, Philadelphia, 2000.

Kozier, B, Erb, G, Blais, K, and Wilkinson, M: Fundamentals of Nursing, ed 5. Addison-Wesley Longman, Inc., Redwood City, CA, 1998.

Lueckenotte, A: Gerontologic Assessment, ed 3. Mosby, St Louis, 1998.

Muecke, MA: Culture and ethnicity. In Craven, RF, and Hirnle, CJ: Fundamentals of Nursing: Human Health and Function. Lippincott, New York, 1992, pp 236–252.

Murray, RB, and Zentner, JP: Nursing Assessment and Health Promotion Strategies through the Lifespan, ed 6. Appleton and Lange, East Norwalk, CT, 1997, p. 47.

Seidel, HM, Ball, JW, Dains, JE, and Benedict, GW: Mosby's Guide to Physical Examination, ed 4. Mosby, St Louis, 1999.

Tanner, JM: Growth at Adolescence. Blackwell, Oxford, England, 1962.

Thomas, CL (ed): Taber's Cyclopedic Medical Dictionary, ed 18. FA Davis, Philadelphia, 1997.

Thompson, JM, McFarland, GK, Hirsch, JE, and Tucken, SM: Mosby's Clinical Nursing, ed 3. Mosby, St Louis, 1993.

U.S. Department of Health and Human Services: Clinical Practice Guideline: Treatment of Pressure Ulcers. USDHHS, Public Health Service, Agency for Health Care Policy and Research, Rockville, MD, December 1994, vol 15.

Bibliography

Barkauskas, V, Stoltenberg-Allen, K, Baumann, L, and Darling-Fisher, C: Health and Physical Assessment, ed 2. Mosby, St Louis, 1998.

Bickley, L, and Hoekelman, R: Bates' Guide to Physical Examination and History Taking, ed 7. Lippincott, Philadelphia, 1999.

Clark, MJ: Nursing in the Community: Dimensions of Community Health Nursing, ed 3. Appleton and Lange, Stamford, CT, 1999.

Edelman, CL, and Mandle, CL: Health Promotion throughout the Lifespan, ed 4. Mosby, St Louis, 1998.

Gallo, JJ, Reichel, W, and Andersen, LM: Handbook of Geriatric Assessment, ed 2. Aspen, Gaithersburg, MD, 1995.

Hogstel, M: Gerontology: Nursing Care of the Older Adult. Delmar, New York, 2001.

Kozier, B, Erb, G, Blais, K, and Wilkinson, JM: Fundamentals of Nursing, ed 5. Addison-Wesley Longman, Redwood City, CA, 1998.

Lueckenotte, AG: Gerontologic Assessment, ed 3. Mosby, St Louis, 1998.

Murray, RB, and Zentner, JP: Nursing Assessment and Health Promotion: Strategies through the Lifespan, ed 6. Appleton and Lange, East Norwalk, CT, 1997.

Seidel, H, Ball, J, Dains, J, and Benedict, GW: Mosby's Guide to Physical Examination, ed 4. Mosby, St Louis, 1999.

Thomas, C (ed): Taber's Cyclopedic Medical Dictionary, ed 18. FA Davis, Philadelphia, 1997.

U.S. Department of Health and Human Services: The Clinician's Handbook of Preventive Services. USDHHS, Alexandria, VA, 1994.

Wong, D, et al: Whaley and Wong's Nursing Care of Infants and Children, ed 6. Mosby, St Louis, 1999.

Index

An f following a page number indicates a figure. A t indicates a table.